# DEMONSTRATIN    ...K
# COMPETENCE 1:
# HEALTHCARE TEACHING

**Ruth Chambers**
**Kay Mohanna**
**Gill Wakley**
**and**
**David Wall**

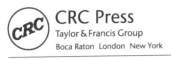

## CRC Press
Taylor & Francis Group
Boca Raton  London  New York

CRC Press is an imprint of the
Taylor & Francis Group, an **informa** business

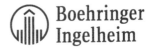

Boehringer
Ingelheim

Provided as a service to medicine by Boehringer Ingelheim

CRC Press
Taylor & Francis Group
6000 Broken Sound Parkway NW, Suite 300
Boca Raton, FL 33487-2742

**Visit the Taylor & Francis Web site at**
**http://www.taylorandfrancis.com**

**and the CRC Press Web site at**
**http://www.crcpress.com**

# Contents

# Preface

As professionals, we should demonstrate our competence in the roles of our daily work. If we are working as teachers in the healthcare professions, either full or part-time, in formal posts such as GP, nurse or staff trainers, or informally such as within healthcare teams, we need to gather evidence that we are staying up to date and maintaining our competence as teachers. In the drive to regulate professionals' standards of practice, everyone must collect and retain information that demonstrates their current competence in their work.

The General Medical Council has asked doctors to start thinking now about how they will collect and keep the information that will show that they should continue to hold a licence to practise as doctors from 2005 onwards. The onus will be on individual doctors to show that they are up to date and fit to practise medicine throughout their careers. It will be doctors who decide for themselves the nature of the information they collect and retain, that best reflects their roles and responsibilities in their everyday work.[1]

Post-registration education and practice (PREP) requirements for nurses were introduced in 1990 and endorsed by the Nursing and Midwifery Council (NMC) in 2002. Nurses have been engaged in portfolio demonstration of learning activity through their PREP requirements since 1995. It requires practitioners to undertake and record their continuing professional development over the three years before they renew their professional registration.[2] Other health professional regulatory bodies are following suit.

This book is one of a series that will guide you through the process, giving you examples and ideas as to how to document your learning, competence, performance or standards of service delivery as a teacher. Other books in the series focus on clinical care rather than teaching.

Chapter 1 explains the link between your personal development plans and local appraisal and, if you are a doctor, the revalidation of your medical registration. Learning and development of your teaching practice that is integral to your personal development plan is central to the evidence you include in your appraisal (and revalidation) portfolio.

The stages of the evidence cycle that we suggest are built upon the underpinning publication:

Chambers R, Wakley G, Field S and Ellis S (2003) *Appraisal for the Apprehensive*. Radcliffe Medical Press, Oxford.

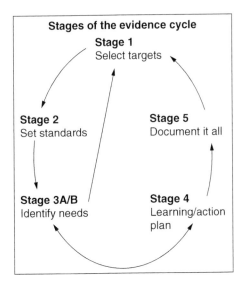

**Stages of the evidence cycle**
**Stage 1**
Select targets

**Stage 2**
Set standards

**Stage 5**
Document it all

**Stage 3A/B**
Identify needs

**Stage 4**
Learning/action plan

Stage 1 is about setting targets or aspirations for good practice. Many of the aspirations we suggest are taken from *Good Medical Practice*[3] or its sister publication, *Good Medical Practice for General Practitioners*,[4] both of which documents are generally applicable to all healthcare professionals. Stage 2 encourages you to set standards for the outcomes of what you plan to learn more about, or outcomes relating to you providing an educational environment in your practice as a clinician and a teacher.

Chapter 2 describes a variety of methods to help you to address Stage 3 of the cycle of evidence, to find out what it is you need to learn about or what gaps there are in the way you work as a teacher. This chapter includes a wide variety of methods that health professionals who also teach might use to identify and document these needs.

Best practice in addressing the giving of informed consent by patients, maintaining confidentiality of patient information and organising responsive complaints processes are all common components of good quality healthcare. They are all also integral to how we work as healthcare teachers. Chapter 3 covers these aspects in depth and provides the first example of cycles of evidence for you to consider adopting or adapting for your own circumstances. The focus of each cycle of evidence is on a standard appraisal format such as one of the 'headings' from *Good Medical Practice*.[3,5] In this chapter examples of cycles of evidence may not be directly related to teaching but give practical examples of methods that can be applied in clinical care or generalised to teaching.

The rest of the book consists of nine chapters that span key aspects of adult learning in a healthcare context. The first part of each chapter gives an introduction to educational theory or practical aspects of teaching. These sections draw on the companion volume to this one: Mohanna K, Wall D and Chambers R (2003) *Teaching Made Easy* (2e). Radcliffe Medical Press, Oxford. The second part of each chapter gives specific teaching examples of cycles of evidence in a similar format to those in Chapter 3.

Overall, you will probably want to choose three or four cycles of evidence each year, considering different aspects of your teaching and clinical practice. You might like this way of learning and service development so much that you build up a bigger bank of evidence of as many as ten cycles in the same year. Whatever your approach, you will want to keep your cycles of evidence as short and simple as possible, so that the documentation itself is a by-product of the learning and action plans you undertake to improve the service you provide, and does not dominate your time and effort at work. Other books in the series are based on the same format of the five stages in the cycle of evidence, setting out key information and examples of evidence for a wide variety of clinical areas.

This approach and style of learning will take a bit of getting used to. Until now, nurses, doctors and other health professionals have not had to prove that they are fit to practise unless the Nursing and Midwifery Council or General Medical Council or other regulatory councils have investigated them for a significant reason such as a patient complaint or significant error. Until recently, most doctors or other health professionals did not evaluate what they learnt or whether they applied it in practice. They did not protect time for learning and reflection among their everyday responsibilities, or target their time and effort on priority topics. Times are changing, and with the introduction of personal development plans and appraisal, health professionals are realising that they must take a more professional approach to learning and document their standards of competence, performance and service delivery, both as teachers and as clinicians. This book helps them to do just that.

**Please note that resources to support this book are provided at http://health.mattersonline.net.**

# References

1   General Medical Council (2003) *A Licence to Practise and Revalidation*. General Medical Council, London. http://www.gmc-uk.org.

2   http://www.nmc-uk.org.

3   General Medical Council (2001) *Good Medical Practice*. General Medical Council, London.

4   Royal College of General Practitioners/General Practitioners Committee (2002) *Good Medical Practice for General Practitioners*. Royal College of General Practitioners, London.

5   Department of Health (2002) *GP Appraisal*. Department of Health, London.

# About the authors

**Ruth Chambers** has been a GP for 20 years. Her previous experience has encompassed a wide range of research and educational activities, including stress and the health of doctors, the quality of healthcare, healthy working, the care of prisoners and those with learning disability, teenagers' contraception, and many other topics.

She is currently a part-time GP, Head of Stoke-on-Trent Teaching Primary Care Trust programme and Professor of Primary Care Development at Staffordshire University. She is the national education lead for the NHS Alliance. Ruth has initiated and run all types of educational initiatives and activities. These have ranged from small group work, to plenary lectures, distance learning programmes, workshops and courses in personal management skills, with audiences of all types of health professionals and occasionally lay audiences.

**Kay Mohanna** is a principal in general practice, a GP trainer and principal lecturer in medical education at Staffordshire University. She is responsible for development and delivery of the Masters in Medical Education, and is lead tutor for the ethics module of the Masters in Primary Care. She has developed and run 'teaching the teachers' courses for consultants, dentists, GPs, physiotherapists, cytologists and other healthcare professional groups and is a co-facilitator on the West Midlands modular GP trainers' course. She is the West Midlands Deanery GP appraisal lead. Her current research interest is in evaluating the process of 'expert review' of teaching practice as a way to increase teaching effectiveness.

**Gill Wakley** started in general practice but transferred to community medicine shortly afterwards and then into public health. A desire for increased contact with patients caused a move back into general practice. She has been heavily involved in learning and teaching throughout her career. She was in a training general practice, became an instructing doctor and a regional assessor in family planning and was, until recently, a senior clinical lecturer with the Primary Care Department at Keele University. Like Ruth, she has run all types of educational initiatives and activities. A visiting professor at Staffordshire University, she now works as a freelance GP, writer and lecturer.

**David Wall** is the deputy regional postgraduate dean in the West Midlands and has been a full-time GP in the same practice for nearly 30 years. He was previously the West Midlands regional adviser in general practice for five years. He runs 'teaching the teachers' educational skills training at basic and advanced levels. He is now responsible for teaching consultants and has taught hundreds of people over the years. His dissertation for the Masters in Medical Education at the University of Dundee included an investigation of doctors' learning needs and styles.

# 1

## Making the link: personal development plans and appraisal

## The nexus of personal development plans, appraisal and revalidation

Learning involves many steps. It includes the acquisition of information, its retention, the ability to retrieve the information when needed and how to use that information for best practice. Demonstrating your learning involves being able to show the steps you have taken. Learning should be lifelong and encompass continuing professional development.

Continuing professional development (CPD) takes time. It makes sense to utilise the time spent by overlapping learning to meet your personal and professional needs with that required for the performance of your role in the health service.

Many health professionals have drawn up a personal development plan (PDP) that is agreed with their local CPD or college tutor. Some health professionals have constructed their PDP in a systematic way and identified the priorities within it, or gathered evidence to demonstrate that what they learnt about was subsequently applied in practice. Tutors do not have a uniform approach to the style and relevance of a health professional's PDP. Some are content that a plan has been drawn up, while others encourage the health professional to develop a systematic approach to identifying and addressing their learning and service needs, in order of importance or urgency.[1]

The new emphasis on health professionals' accountability to the public has given the PDP a higher profile and shown that it may be used in other ways. The medical education establishment and NHS management argue about the balance between its alternative uses. Educationalists view a PDP as a tool to encourage health professionals to plan their own learning activities. The management view is of a tool allowing quality assurance of the health professional's performance. Doctors, striving to improve the quality of the care that they deliver to patients, want to use a PDP to guide them on their way, perhaps towards postgraduate awards of universities or the quality awards of the Royal College of General Practitioners (RCGP). These quality awards are built around the standards of excellence to which members of the primary care team should aspire, such as within the Quality Team Development award.[2]

# Your personal development plan

Your PDP will be an integral part of your future appraisal and, if you are a doctor, your revalidation portfolio to demonstrate your fitness to practise.
    Your initial plan should:

- identify your gaps or weaknesses in knowledge, skills or attitudes
- specify topics for learning as a result of changes: in your role, responsibilities, the organisation in which you work
- link into the learning needs of others in your workplace or team of colleagues
- tie in with the service development priorities of your practice, the primary care organisation (PCO) or the NHS as a whole
- describe how you identified your learning needs
- set your learning needs and associated goals in order of importance and urgency
- justify your selection of learning goals
- describe how you will achieve your goals and over what time period
- describe how you will evaluate learning outcomes.

Each year you will continue or revise your PDP. It should demonstrate how you carried out your learning and evaluation plans, show that you have learnt what you set out to do (or why it was modified) and how you applied your new learning in practice. In addition, you will find that you have new priorities and fresh learning needs as circumstances change.
    The main task is to capture what you have learnt, in a way that suits you. Then you can look back at what you have done and:

- reflect on it later, to decide to learn more, or to make changes as a result, and identify further needs
- demonstrate to others that you are fit to practise or work through:
    - what you have done
    - what you have learnt
    - what changes you have made as a result
    - the standards of work you have achieved and are maintaining
    - how you monitor your performance at work
- use it to show how your personal learning fits in with the requirements of your practice or the NHS, and other people's personal and professional development plans.

Organise all the evidence of your learning into a continuing professional development portfolio of some sort. It is up to you how you keep this record of your learning. Examples are:

- *an ongoing learning journal* in which you draw up and describe your plan, record how you determined your needs and prioritised them, report why you attended particular educational meetings or courses and what you got out of them as well as the continuing cycle of review, making changes and evaluating them
- *an A4 file* with lots of plastic sleeves into which you build up a systematic record of your educational activities in line with your plan
- *a box*: chuck in everything to do with your learning plan as you do it and sort it out into a sensible order every few months with a good review once a year.

# The context of appraisal and revalidation for doctors

Appraisal and revalidation are based on the same sources of information – presented in the same structure as the headings set out in the General Medical Council (GMC) guidance in *Good Medical Practice*.[3] The two processes perform different functions. Whereas revalidation involves an assessment against a standard of fitness to practise medicine, appraisal is concerned with the doctor's professional development within his or her working environment and the needs of the organisation for which the doctor works.

Appraisal is a formative and developmental process that is being introduced by the Departments of Health for all general practitioners (GPs) and hospital consultants working in the NHS across the UK. While the details of the appraisal system vary for consultants and GPs and for each of the countries, the educational principles remain the same. The aims of the appraisal system are to give doctors an opportunity to discuss and receive regular feedback on their previous and continuing performance and identify education and development needs.

The drive to introduce formal appraisals came initially as part of the programme to introduce clinical governance across the NHS as laid out in the 1998 consultation document *A First Class Service*.[4] Momentum was gained with the publication of *Supporting Doctors, Protecting Patients* (1999) in England which outlined a set of proposals to help prevent doctors from developing problems.[5] Appraisal was at the heart of the proposals as:

a positive process to give someone feedback on their performance, to chart their continuing progress and to identify development needs. It is a forward looking process essential for the developmental and educational planning needs of an individual. *Assessment* is the process of measuring progress against agreed criteria ... It is not the primary aim of appraisal to scrutinise doctors to see if they are performing poorly but rather to help them consolidate and improve on good performance aiming towards excellence.[5]

The document went on to suggest that appraisal should be made comprehensive and compulsory for doctors working in the NHS and form part of a future revalidation system.

In addition, appraisal should also address other areas of particular importance to the individual doctor. A standardised approach has been developed which utilises approved documentation. This should ensure that information from a variety of NHS employers is recorded consistently. The format of the paperwork is slightly different for consultants and GPs.

Appraisal must be a positive, formative and developmental process to support high quality patient care and improve clinical standards. Appraisal is different from, but linked to, revalidation.[6] Revalidation is the process whereby doctors will be regularly required to demonstrate that they are fit to practise. Appraisal feeds into this by contributing to the information that a doctor supplies for the revalidation process. Appraisal will provide a regular, structured recording system for documenting progress towards revalidation and identifying needs as part of the doctor's PDP. Both the NHS appraisal and the revalidation structures are based on the same seven headings set out in the GMC's guidance *Good Medical Practice.*[3] The GMC claims, therefore, that 'five appraisals equals revalidation'.[6] The GMC has also pledged that doctors not taking part in appraisal in a managed system will be able to provide their own information for revalidation, providing this evidence meets the same criteria as in *Good Medical Practice* (the independent route).

Appraisal is, however, a two-way process. Not only time, but also resources will be needed to make appraisal systems successful. In addition, appraisal will identify issues that will require extra investment by the NHS in the educational and organisational infrastructure.

Appraisal and revalidation processes are being increasingly integrated. The PDP is a central part of the appraisal documentation, which will in turn be included in the portfolio of information available for revalidation. It seems that the evolution will continue so that revalidation is met by supporting the appraisal documentation with additional documents about clinical governance activity and CPD. These supporting documents will be a mix of subjective and objective information that will include doctors' self-assessment of their performance and other work-based assessment.

The revalidation and appraisal processes need to be quality assured to be able to demonstrate that they can protect the public from poor or under-performing doctors. Such quality assurance will relate to the appraisers, their training and support, as well as systems to examine the quality of evidence in the documentation relating to a doctor's performance and outcomes of their PDP. You should regard your PDP and supporting documentation as central to the way in which you can show, to anyone who requires you to do so, that your performance as a doctor is acceptable and that you are trying to improve, or striving for excellence.

# Demonstrating the standards of your practice as a health professional

Doctors must be able to meet the standards of *Good Medical Practice* with a record of their own performance in their revalidation portfolio if they want to retain a licence to practise.[3] The nine key headings of expected standards of practice (*see* Box 1.1) for all GPs working in England are just as relevant to all health professionals.

---

**Box 1.1:**   Key headings of expected standards of practice for GPs working in England

1  *Good professional practice.* This relates to clinical care, keeping records (including writing reports and keeping colleagues informed), access and availability, treatment in emergencies and making effective use of resources.
2  *Maintaining good medical practice.* This includes keeping up to date and maintaining your performance.
3  *Relationships with patients.* This encompasses providing information about your services, maintaining trust, avoiding discrimination and prejudice against patients, relating well to patients and apologising if things go wrong.
4  *Working with colleagues.* This relates to working with colleagues, working in teams, referring patients and accepting posts.
5  *Teaching and training, appraising and assessing.* You may be in a position to teach or train colleagues or students, and appraise or assess peers, employees or students.
6  *Probity* includes providing true information about your services, honesty in financial and commercial dealings, and providing references.
7  *Health* can include how you overcome or compensate for health problems in yourself, or help with or address health problems in other doctors.
8  *Research.* Conducting research in an ethical manner.
9  *Management.* The section on management concerns any responsibility GPs or other health professionals have for management outside the practice. GPs or other health professionals might wish to include management responsibilities that cross the interface between their practice and primary care organisation (PCO).

---

The appraisal paperwork for GPs working in England, Scotland, Wales and Northern Ireland has been individualised by each country. The English version, for example, includes two extra sections to those of hospital consultants, management and research. The Scottish version focuses on core categories in preparation for revalidation of prescribing, referrals and peer review, clinical audit, significant event analysis and communication skills, summary of any complaints and other feedback. There is no standard format of appraisal for non-doctors in the NHS – but any of the medical versions alluded to here may be adapted.

## The evidence cycle

The stages of the evidence cycle for demonstrating your standards of practice or competence and any necessary improvements in your teaching practice are given in Figure 1.1. The stages of the evidence cycle are common to all the various areas of expertise considered in this book and will be followed in each chapter.

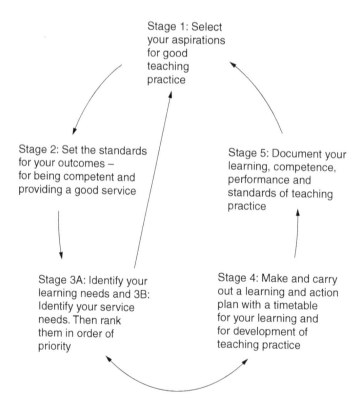

**Figure 1.1:**   Stages of the evidence cycle.

Although the five stages are shown in sequence here, in practice you would expect to move backwards and forwards from stage to stage, because of new information or a modification of your earlier ideas. New information might accrue when educational research is published which affects your teaching methods or standards, or a critical incident or patient complaint might occur which causes you and others to think anew about the way teaching is carried out in your practice. The arrows in Figure 1.1 show that you might reset your target or aspirations for good practice having undertaken exercises to identify what you need to learn or determine whether there are deficiencies in your teaching practice.

We suggest that you demonstrate your competence in focused areas of your day-to-day work by completing several cycles of evidence drawn from a variety of clinical or other areas each year, with at least one cycle of evidence from each of the main headings of *Good Medical Practice* over a five-year cycle.[3] By demonstrating your standards of practice around the main sections of *Good Medical Practice*, you will document your competence and performance for your revalidation portfolio in the same format as that required for your appraisal paperwork.

As you start to collate information around this five-stage cycle, discuss any problems about your teaching practice with colleagues, experts in this area, tutors, etc. You want to develop a wide range and depth of evidence so that you can show that you are competent in your day-to-day general work as well as for any special areas of expertise.

Professional competence is the first area of concern in *Good Medical Practice*.[3] You should be able to demonstrate that you can maintain a satisfactory standard of care most of the time in your everyday work. Some of the time you will be brilliant, of course! Celebrate those moments. On other occasions, you or others will be critical of your performance and feel that you could have done much better. Reflect on those episodes to learn from them.

## Stage 1: Select your aspirations for good practice

By adopting or adapting descriptions of what an 'excellent' GP or other health professional should be aiming for, you are defining the standards of practice for which all should be aiming. The medical Royal Colleges have interpreted *Good Medical Practice* in various ways for the specialities of their own members.[3] For example, *Good Medical Practice for General Practitioners* describes the standards of practice that should be achieved by 'excellent' or 'unacceptable' GPs.[7] Their definition of excellence is being 'consistently good'.[2]

This consistency is a critical factor in considering competence and performance too (*see* page 15). The documents that you collect in your evidence cycles must reflect consistency over time and in different circumstances, for example with various types of learners. This will show that you have not only performed well on one occasion or for one type of baseline assessment, but also sustained your performance over time and under different conditions.

# Stage 2: Set the standards for your outcomes – for being competent and providing a good service

Outcomes might include:

- a tutorial plan
- mastery of a new skill as a teacher
- a teaching strategy that is implemented
- learner feedback
- evaluation of teaching programmes.

The level at which you should be performing depends on your expertise and experience and will be specific to you. You would be expected to demonstrate progress, year on year, and are not expected to be expert from the word go.

You could incorporate into your standards or outcomes those components specified by universities at a national level as part of their Masters' Frameworks for their postgraduate awards. The national Masters' Framework consists of eight components that shape the individual postgraduate award programme outcomes and the learning outcomes of the individual modules for the postgraduate awards. The eight components are shown in Box 1.2. You could set out your CPD work in the portfolio you are assembling for revalidation and your annual appraisals in this format. This would help you to document your professional development to date in a form that can be readily 'accredited for prior experiential learning' (APEL) by universities (contact your local universities if you want more information about this process). You might then be

---

**Box 1.2:**    The eight components of the Masters' Frameworks for postgraduate awards

1    Analysis
2    Problem solving
3    Knowledge and understanding
4    Reflection
5    Communication
6    Learning
7    Application
8    Enquiry

given credits for learning against an intended postgraduate award. It would save you from duplicating work as well as speeding your progress through the award.

If you have information or data about your practice showing that it was substandard or that you were not competent, you might simply choose to exclude that from your portfolio. However, you will be able to show that you have learnt more by reviewing mistakes or negative episodes. It is better to include everything of relevance, then go on to demonstrate how you addressed the gaps in your performance and made sustained improvements.

You will need to protect the confidentiality of patients, colleagues and learners as necessary when you collect data. The GMC will be seeing the contents of a doctor's revalidation portfolio if it is one of those sampled. You will probably also submit or share the documentation for appraisal and maybe use it for reviews with colleagues or the PCO. Make sure that individual learners cannot be identified from your portfolio.

# Stage 3: Identify your learning and service needs in your practice or primary care organisation and rank them in order of priority[1]

The type and depth of documentation you need to gather will encompass:

- the context in which you work
- your knowledge and skills in relation to any particular role or responsibility of your current post.

The extent of expertise you should possess will depend on your level of responsibility for a particular function or task. You may be the sole trainer in a practice, or be part of a team responsible for undergraduate students. You may be personally responsible for a function or task, or you may contribute or delegate responsibility for it. Your learning needs should take into account your aspirations for the future too – personal or career development for you, or improvements in the way you manage teaching in your practice. Look at Chapter 2 for more ideas on how you will identify your learning or service development needs.

Group and summarise your development needs from the exercises you have carried out. Grade them according to the priority you set. You may put one at a higher priority because it fits in with service development needs established in the business plan of the trust or practice, or put another lower because it does not fit in with other activities that your organisation has in their current development plan for the next 12 months. If you have identified a development need by several different methods of assessment, or if it is a common theme in learner feedback, then it will have a higher priority than something only identified once. Notify the development needs you have identified to those responsible for agreeing and implementing the development plans of the trust and/or practice.

Look back at your aspirations and standards set out in Stages 1 and 2. Match your learning or service development needs with one or more of these standards, or others that you have set yourself.

# Stage 4: Make and carry out a learning and action plan with a timetable for your personal and service development

If you have not identified any learning needs for yourself or the service as a whole, you should omit Stage 4 and tidy up the presentation of your evidence for inclusion in your portfolio as at the end of Stage 5.

Think about whether:

- you have defined your learning objectives – what you need to learn to be able to attain the standards and outcomes you have described in Stage 2
- you can justify spending time and effort on the topics you prioritised in Stage 3. Is the topic important enough to your work, your learners or the NHS as a whole? Does the event occur sufficiently often to warrant the time spent?
- the time and resources for learning about that topic or making the associated changes to your teaching are available. Check that you are not trying to do too much too quickly, or you will become discouraged
- learning about that topic will make a tangible difference to the way you teach
- and how one topic fits in with other topics you have identified to learn more about. Have you achieved a good balance across your areas of work or between your personal aspirations and the basic requirements of the service?

Decide on what method of learning is most appropriate for your task or role or the standards you are expecting to attain or sustain. You may have already identified your preferred learning style – but read up on this elsewhere if you are unsure.[8]

Describe how you will carry out your learning tasks and what you will do by a specified time. State how your learning will be applied and how and when it will be evaluated. Build in some staging posts so that you do not suddenly get to the end of 12 months and discover that you have only done half of your plan.

Your action plan should also include your role in remedying any gaps in your teaching practice that you identified in Stage 3 and that are within the remit of your responsibility.

## Stage 5: Document your learning, competence, performance and standards of service delivery

You might choose to document that you have attained your defined outcomes by repeating the learning needs assessment that you started with. You could record your increased confidence and competence in dealing with situations that you previously avoided or performed inadequately.

You might incorporate your assessment of what has been gained in a study of another area that overlaps.

# Preparing your portfolio[9–11]

The portfolio of supporting documents that accumulates as you carry out your learning might form the basis of professional revalidation or recertification. This has been the case for some time under post-registration education and practice (PREP) requirements for nurses. Introduced in 1990, PREP was again endorsed by the Nursing and Midwifery Council (NMC) in 2002 and requires practitioners to undertake and record their CPD over the three years prior to renewal of their professional registration.[12]

The NMC regularly audits a sample of nurses who are required to provide such evidence of their learning activity and the relevance of this learning to their work. Similarly the GMC has said that the basis of revalidation for doctors will be five 'successful' appraisals; the outcome of each will be a PDP showing learning under the headings of *Good Medical Practice*.

Use your portfolio of evidence of what you have learnt and your standards of practice to:

- identify significant experiences to serve as important sources of learning
- reflect on the learning that arose from those experiences
- demonstrate learning in practice
- analyse and identify further learning needs and ways in which these needs can be met.

Your documentation might include all sorts of things, not just learner feedback – although that makes a good start. It might include reports of educational activities attended, statements of your roles and responsibilities, copies of publications you have read and critically appraised, and reports of your work.

You could incorporate observations of your teaching by others (peer review), evaluations of you observing other colleagues and how their practice differs from yours, descriptions of self-improvements, a video of a tutorial or teaching session with a self-critique, materials that demonstrate your skills to others, or products of your input or learning – a new teaching visual aid for example. Box 1.3 gives a list of material you might include in your portfolio.

---

**Box 1.3:**   Possible contents of a portfolio

- Videotaped teaching sessions with self-critique
- Learner feedback
- Results of peer review of teaching sessions
- Anonymised reports from appraisal sessions you have facilitated for others
- Lesson plans
- Commentaries on published educational literature or books
- Records of complaints from learners with learning points
- Formal evaluation of teaching programmes
- Training sessions you have attended with commentary on how you benefited or implemented change as a result
- Visual aids you have developed
- PowerPoint presentations that you have given (CD, floppy disk)

---

Once you are preparing to submit the portfolio for a discussion with a colleague (for example, at an appraisal) or assessment (for example, for a university postgraduate award or revalidation) write a self-assessment of your previous action plan. You might integrate your self-assessment into your personal development plan to show what you have achieved and what gaps you have still to address. Decide where are you now and where you want to be in one, three or five years' time. Select items from your portfolio for inclusion for each part of the documentation – you might have one compartment of your portfolio per speciality topic or section heading from *Good Medical Practice*.[3]

Make sure all references are included and the documentation in your portfolio is as accurate and complete as possible. Organise how you have shown your learning steps and your standards of practice so that it is indexed and cross-referenced to the relevant sections of the paperwork. Discuss the contents of your portfolio with a colleague or a mentor to gain other people's perspectives of your work and look for blind-spots.

# Include evidence of your competence from other sources

You may have particular expertise or a special interest in a teaching field. Whatever your role or responsibility or expertise, your portfolio should include examples of evidence that show that you are competent, and that you have a consistently good performance in your speciality area.[13] You may have parallel appraisals that you can include from your employer – for example, the university if you have a formal teaching post, or the result of the practice accreditation visit for general dental practice trainers.

When you gather evidence of your performance as a teacher, try to document as many aspects of your work at one time as you can, so that one piece of supporting information covers as many of the key headings from *Good Medical Practice* (*see* page 5) as possible.[3] When you are identifying what you need to learn, or gaps in your teaching practice, make sure that you involve patients and show how you interact with the team. This gives you evidence about 'relationships with patients' and 'working with colleagues' as well as the teaching area you are focusing on or auditing.

# Link your cycles of evidence to service developments rewarded by the new General Medical Services (GMS) Contract or Personal Medical Services (PMS) arrangements

If you work in general practice, the areas within the primary care quality framework will probably be the ones that you prioritise in your PDP when looking at your service development needs.[14] The four main components of the quality framework are all relevant to your personal and professional development in respect of your clinical care rather than your teaching. The clinical and organisational standards may be those which you are aiming for in Stage 2 of the evidence cycle (*see* Figure 1.1). Achieving the standards in the quality framework will follow on from the descriptions of an excellent health professional (Stage 1). Identifying personal learning needs and service development needs, that is, the gaps between baseline and specified standards in the quality framework, is in Stage 3. Making and carrying out your personal learning plan and service improvements in line with patients' experience is in Stage 4. Producing the documentation that shows you have attained the clinical or organisational standards required for core or additional services and responded to patients' views is in Stage 5.

# References

1   Wakley G, Chambers R and Field S (2000) *Continuing Professional Development in Primary Care.* Radcliffe Medical Press, Oxford.

2   Quality Team Development, Royal College of General Practitioners, London – see details on www.rcgp.org.uk/qtd/index.asp.

3   General Medical Council (2001) *Good Medical Practice.* General Medical Council, London.

4   Department of Health (1998) *A First Class Service.* Department of Health, London.

5   Department of Health (1999) *Supporting Doctors, Protecting Patients.* Department of Health, London.

6   General Medical Council (2003) *Licence to Practise and Revalidation for Doctors.* General Medical Council, London. www.revalidationuk.info.

7   Royal College of General Practitioners/General Practitioners' Committee (2002) *Good Medical Practice for General Practitioners.* Royal College of General Practitioners, London.

8   Mohanna K, Wall D and Chambers R (2003) *Teaching Made Easy: a manual for health professionals* (2e). Radcliffe Medical Press, Oxford.

9   Royal College of General Practitioners (1993) *Portfolio-based Learning in General Practice.* Occasional Paper 63, Royal College of General Practitioners, London.

10  Challis M (1999) AMEE Medical education guide No 11 (revised): portfolio-based learning and assessment in medical education. *Medical Teacher.* **21 (4)**: 370–86.

11  Chambers C, Wakley G, Field S and Ellis S (2003) *Appraisal for the Apprehensive.* Radcliffe Medical Press, Oxford.

12  http://www.nmc-uk.org.

13  www.gpwsi.org.

14  General Practitioners' Committee/The NHS Confederation (2003) *New GMS Contract. Investing in general practice.* General Practitioners' Committee, London.

# 2

## Practical ways to identify your learning and service needs as part of the documentation of your competence and performance as a clinician and a teacher

## Setting standards to show that you are competent

Doctors 'must be committed to lifelong learning and be responsible for maintaining the medical knowledge and clinical and team skills necessary for the provision of quality care'.[1]

Nurses, allied health professionals and others have similar responsibilities.

You could make a good start by describing your roles and responsibilities. This will help you to define what your competence should be now, or what competence you are hoping to attain, for instance accreditation of the practice for training status. Once you have your definition, you can recognise whether you have, or lack in some part, the necessary competence and what you will need to work towards. If there are no accepted descriptions of competence in the area you are focusing on, then you will have to start from scratch. You might compile your description from guidelines such as regional criteria for a training practice. Usually you can find guidance about competency from specialist sources such the various Royal Colleges or universities.

A good definition of competence is someone who is: 'able to perform the tasks and roles required to the expected standard'.[2]

You will need to describe the standards expected in the range of tasks and roles you undertake and reference the source of standard setting. If professionals, or their organisations, are the only people involved in setting those standards, consider whether you should amend or extend the standards, tasks or roles by considering other perspectives such as those of students, patients or the NHS as a whole.

There is a difference between being competent, and performing in a consistently competent manner. You need to be motivated to perform consistently well and enabled to do so with efficient systems and sufficient resources. You will require sufficient numbers of other competent doctors or staff and available infrastructure such as teaching aids and resources.[3]

Choose methods in Stage 3 (*see* Chapter 1) to demonstrate your standards of performance and identify any learning needs that span different topic areas, to reduce duplication and maximise the usefulness of your learning. Collecting evidence of more than one aspect of your competence or performance cuts down the overall amount of work underpinning your PDP or included in your appraisal portfolio.

Use several methods to identify your learning needs and/or gaps in your teaching development or delivery, so that you validate the findings of one method by another. No one method will give you reliable information about the gaps in your knowledge, skills or attitudes or everyday service. Does what you think about your performance match with what learners, others in the team or patients think of how you practise in your everyday work? It is particularly difficult to determine what it is you 'don't know you don't know' by yourself, yet it is vital that you identify and rectify those gaps. Other people may be able to tell you quite readily what you need to learn. Colleagues from different disciplines could usefully comment on any shortfalls in how your work interfaces with theirs.

Learners for whom you are no longer responsible and are therefore no longer under any obligation to you could tell you whether any aspects of the way you teach are off-putting or inappropriate. There may be information you could gather from peer review that could point out those gaps in your knowledge or skills of which you were previously unaware.

Determine what it is that you 'don't know you don't know' by:

* asking learners and ex-learners
* comparing your performance against best practice or that of peers
* comparing your performance against objectives in university standards
* asking colleagues from different disciplines about shortfalls in how your work interfaces with theirs.

# Stage 3A: Identify your learning needs – how you can find out if you need to be better at doing your job

You may decide to use a few selected methods to gather baseline evidence of your performance, focused on your specific area of expertise. You may target other topics or areas at the same time that are relevant to the various sections of the GMC's booklet *Good Medical Practice*.[4] For this type of combined assessment, you might use several of the methods described in this chapter such as:

- constructive feedback from learners, peers or patients
- 360° feedback of your teaching
- self-assessment, or review by others, using a rating scale to assess your skills and attitudes
- comparison with protocols and guidelines for checking how well procedures are followed
- audit: various types and applications
- significant event audit relating to teaching and training
- eliciting learners' or patients' views such as satisfaction surveys
- a SWOT (strengths, weaknesses, opportunities and threats) or SCOT (strengths, challenges, opportunities and threats) analysis
- reading and reflecting
- educational review.

Several of these methods will also be useful for identifying development needs – you can look at the gaps identified from both the personal and service perspectives at the same time using the same method.

## Seek feedback

Find colleagues who will give you constructive feedback about your teaching performance and practice. The golden rule for giving constructive feedback is to give positive praise of things that have been well done first. Sometimes colleagues launch straight in to criticise faults when asked for their views. The Pendleton model of giving feedback is widely used in the health setting (*see* Box 2.1).[5]

**Box 2.1:**   The Pendleton model of giving feedback[5]

1   The learner goes first and performs the activity.
2   Questions clarify any facts.
3   The learner says what they thought was done well.
4   The teacher says what they thought was done well.
5   The learner says what could be improved upon.
6   The teacher says what could be improved upon.
7   Both discuss ideas for improvements in a helpful and constructive manner.

Sticking to this model will help identify those areas you perform well in as well as those you need to improve.

## 360° feedback

This collects together perceptions from a number of different participants as shown in Figure 2.1.

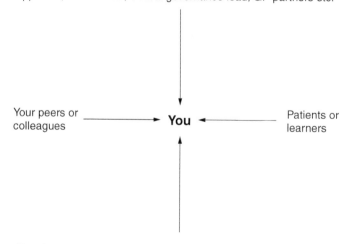

**Figure 2.1:**   360° feedback.

The wider the spread of people giving feedback, the more rounded the picture. You should aim to give a feedback questionnaire to at least three people in each of the groups above. An independent person then collects and collates the questionnaires and discusses the results with the individual. Computerised versions are available from commercial companies.[6] The main disadvantage of this method is that it can sometimes be spoilt by malicious comments against which individuals cannot readily defend themselves.

# Self-assess or gain another person's perspective of your standard of teaching practice

You might describe any aspect of your teaching practice as statements (A to G as in Box 2.2) for you to self-assess, or others to give you feedback or comments by marking the extent to which they agree on the linear scales below. You could modify the descriptions of an excellent GP in *Good Medical Practice for General Practitioners* as we have done in relating statements about teaching

---

**Box 2.2:** Marking grid: circle the number which represents your views or feelings about each statement – complete the grid on more than one occasion and compare results over time

A   I consistently treat learners politely and with consideration.

STRONGLY AGREE                          to                          STRONGLY DISAGREE
1-----------------2-----------------3-----------------4-----------------5-----------------6

B   I am aware of how my personal beliefs could affect the way I teach, and take care not to impose my own beliefs and values.

STRONGLY AGREE                          to                          STRONGLY DISAGREE
1-----------------2-----------------3-----------------4-----------------5-----------------6

C   I always treat all learners equally and ensure that some are not favoured at the expense of others.

STRONGLY AGREE                          to                          STRONGLY DISAGREE
1-----------------2-----------------3-----------------4-----------------5-----------------6

D   I try to maintain a relationship with the learner when a mistake has occurred.

STRONGLY AGREE                          to                          STRONGLY DISAGREE
1-----------------2-----------------3-----------------4-----------------5-----------------6

E   I always obtain informed consent to involve patients in teaching.

STRONGLY AGREE                          to                          STRONGLY DISAGREE

1-----------------2-----------------3-----------------4-----------------5-----------------6
F   I usually involve learners in decisions about the teaching programme.

STRONGLY AGREE                          to                          STRONGLY DISAGREE
1-----------------2-----------------3-----------------4-----------------5-----------------6

G   I always respect the right of learners to determine the extent of their participation.

STRONGLY AGREE                          to                          STRONGLY DISAGREE
1-----------------2-----------------3-----------------4-----------------5-----------------6

skills in Box 2.2 to consultation skills.[7] For instance, if statement A is: 'I consistently treat learners politely and with consideration', you could self-assess the extent to which you agree.[7] Alternatively, you could ask colleagues or learners to fill in the assessment form. Objective feedback from external assessment is usually more reliable than your own self-assessment when you may have blind-spots about your own performance. As you become more con-fident in this method of reviewing your competence, you might emphasise how consistent you are in your application of good practice – so in the statements in Box 2.2 we have sometimes included 'consistently', 'always' or 'usually'. You can set your own challenges. If you have a mentor or a 'buddy' in the practice with whom you learn, you might discuss and reflect on the completed marking grids with him or her.

## Compare your performance against protocols or guidelines relating to teaching

Are you familiar with all the protocols or guidelines that are used by others? You might determine your learning needs and those of other practice team members by piling all the protocols or guidelines that exist in your practice in a big heap and rationalising them so that you have a common set across the practice. Working as a team you can compare your own knowledge and usual teaching practice with others and with protocols or guidelines.

Alternatively, you might compare your own practice against a protocol or guideline that is generally accepted at a national or local level. You could audit the standard of your practice to find out how often you adhere to such a protocol or guideline, and if you can justify why you deviate from the recommendations.

## Audit

Audit is:

the method used by health professionals to assess, evaluate, and improve the care of patients in a systematic way, to enhance their health and quality of life.[8]

The five steps of the audit cycle are shown in Box 2.3.

Performance or practice is often broken down for the purposes of audit into the three aspects of structure, process and outcome. Structural audits might concern resources such as equipment, premises, skills, people, etc. Process audits focus on what happens with the learner: for instance, teaching programmes and tutorial strategy. Audits of outcomes consider the impact of teaching on

---

**Box 2.3:** The five steps of the audit cycle

1 Describe the criteria and standards you are trying to achieve.
2 Measure your current performance of how well you are providing care or services in an objective way.
3 Compare your performance against criteria and standards.
4 Identify the need for change – to performance, adjustment of criteria or standards, resources, available data.
5 Make any required changes as necessary and re-audit later.

---

the learner and might include learner satisfaction or improvements in service provision of the learner as healthcare provider. You might look at any aspects of quality of the structure, process and outcome of teaching – focusing on access, equity, efficiency, economy, effectiveness for individual learners etc.[8]

Set standards for your performance, find out how you are doing, search to find out best practice, make the changes and then re-audit your teaching in the future.

## Significant event audit

Think of an incident where you or a learner were involved in a significant event and how you used it as a learning opportunity. This might be a dysfunctional tutorial, an avoidable side-effect from medication prescribed by your trainee, or an angry outburst in public by you or the learner. You can review the case and reflect on the sequence of events that led to that critical event occurring. It is likely that there were a multitude of factors leading up to that significant event. How did you respond to it? What learning opportunities did you take from it? Did you shy away from bringing it up with the learner or did you seize the opportunity it presented? The steps of a significant event audit are shown in Box 2.4.

---

**Box 2.4:** Steps of a significant event audit

• *Step 1*: Describe who was involved, what time of day, what the task/activity was, the context and any other relevant information.
• *Step 2*: Reflect on the effects of the event on the participants and the professionals involved.
• *Step 3*: Discuss the reasons for the event or situation arising with other colleagues, review case notes or other records.

*continued overleaf*

---

- *Step 4*: Decide how you or others might have behaved differently. Describe your options for how the procedures at work might be changed to minimise or eliminate the chances of the event recurring.
- *Step 5*: Plan changes that are needed, how they will be implemented, who will be responsible for what and when, what further training or resources are required. Then carry out the changes.
- *Step 6*: Re-audit later to see whether changes to procedures or new knowledge and skills are having the desired effects. Give feedback to the practice team.

# An assessment by an external body

This is a traditional way of showing that you are competent by taking and passing an examination. It is a good way of testing recalled knowledge in a written or oral examination, or establishing how you behave in a clinical situation on the day of a practical examination, but not much good for measuring anything else. A summative examination (i.e. done at the end of a course of study) gives a measure of your learning up to that date.

You might undertake an objective test of your clinical knowledge and skills. Examples in clinical areas include a computer-based test in the form of multiple-choice questions and patient management problems such as in the RCGP's phased evaluation programme (PEP) CD ROMs (email pep@rcgp-scotland.org.uk) or the Apollo programme available from BMJ Publishing.[9] Various other organisations give multiple-choice questionnaires that you can complete on paper or online and record in your portfolio.[10,11]

The RCGP's series of quality awards provide external assessment – Membership by Assessment of Performance, Fellowship by Assessment, Quality Team Development, etc. Trained assessors will give feedback to individual doctors or practice teams about their performance compared with set standards and their peers. The Quality Assurance Agency inspects the quality of universities' degree courses.

In teaching there are increasing numbers of postgraduate programmes in teaching practice such as Masters in Medical Education awards and 'teaching the teachers' courses. Degree courses have summative assessment processes and many also use self-assessment or peer review to allow feedback on practice.

## Eliciting the views of patients or learners

Part of meeting the criteria for relationships with patients in *Good Medical Practice*[4] might be to assess patients' or learners' satisfaction with:

*   you
*   your practice
*   their role or involvement in teaching.

Avoid surveys where questions are relatively superficial or biased. A more specific enquiry should uncover particular elements of patients' dissatisfaction, which will be more useful if you are trying to identify your learning needs. Use a well-validated patient questionnaire, instead of risking producing your own version with ambiguities and flaws, such as the General Practice Assessment Questionnaire (GPAQ)[12] or the Doctors' Interpersonal Skills Questionnaire (DISQ).[13] Many doctors and practice teams have used these patient survey methods, providing a bank of data against which to compare your performance.

Other sources of feedback from patients might be obtained through suggestion boxes for patients to contribute comments, or the practice team recording all patients' suggestions and complaints however trivial, looking for patterns in the comments received.

There will be learning to be had from every complaint – even if the complaint does not have any substance, there should be something to learn about the shortfall in communication between you and the complainant.

The evolution of the 'expert patient programme' should mean that there is a pool of well-informed patients with chronic conditions who can contribute their insights into what you (or the service) need to learn from a patient's perspective.[14]

## Strengths, weaknesses (or challenges), opportunities and threats (SWOT or SCOT) analysis

You can undertake a SWOT (or SCOT) analysis of your own teaching perform-ance or that of your practice team or practice organisation, working it out on your own, or with a workmate or mentor, or with a group of colleagues. Brainstorm the strengths, weaknesses (or challenges), opportunities and threats of your role or circumstances.

Strengths and weaknesses (or challenges) of your roles might relate to your clinical knowledge or skills, experience, expertise, decision making, com-munication skills, interprofessional relationships, political skills, timekeeping, organisational skills, teaching skills, or research skills. Strengths and weak-nesses (or challenges) of the practice organisation might relate to most of these aspects as well as the way resources are allocated, overall efficiency and the degree to which the practice is patient- or learner-centred.

Opportunities might relate to your unexploited experience or potential strengths, expected changes in the NHS, or resources for which you might bid. For example, you might build on your teaching of undergraduates and aim to become accredited for training.

Threats will include factors and circumstances that prevent you from achieving your aims for personal, professional and practice development or service improvements. They might be to do with your health, turnover in the practice team, or time-limited investment by the PCO.

List the important factors in your SWOT (or SCOT) analysis in order of priority through discussion with colleagues and independent people from outside your practice. Draw up goals and a timed action plan for you or the practice team to follow.

# Informal conversations – in the corridor, over coffee

You learn such a lot when chatting with colleagues at coffee time or over a meal and can become aware of your learning or service development needs at these times. The trainers' workshop for example is a good place to share ideas and listen to what other teachers are up to. This is when you realise that other people are doing things differently from you and if they seem to be doing it better and achieving more, you can challenge yourself to decide if this matter could be one of your blind-spots. Note down your thoughts before you forget them so that you can reflect on them later.

Online discussion groups may provide another source of informal exchanges with colleagues. If you find this difficult to start with, you might 'lurk', viewing the comments and views of other people until you feel confident enough to contribute. Record any observations that you find useful and reflect on how they might inform your own practice.

# Observe your work environment and role

Observation could be informal and opportunistic, or more systematic, working through a structured checklist. One method of self-assessment might be to audiotape yourself at work dealing with learners (after obtaining learners' informed consent). Listen to the tape afterwards to appraise your communication and consultation skills – on your own or with a friend or colleague. If you have access to video equipment, you might use this instead.

Look at the equipment in your practice or library. Do you know how to operate it properly? Assess yourself connecting up the data projector and lap-top computer and developing PowerPoint skills for lectures, or ask some-one to watch you operate the equipment and give you feedback about your performance.

Analyse the various roles and responsibilities of your current posts. Compare your level of expertise against national standards such as in the Knowledge and Skills Framework for England from the Department of Health or a job evaluation framework as part of the Agenda for Change initiative.[15,16] Deter-mine if you can meet the requirements, or, if not, what deficiencies need to be made good.

You might combine one of the methods of identifying your learning needs already described such as an audit or SWOT analysis and apply it to 'observing your work environment or role', describing your relationship with learners and other members of the multidisciplinary team for example, or reviewing how their roles and responsibilities interface with yours.

## Reading and reflecting

Get into the habit of reading educational journals, and when reading articles reflect on what the key messages mean for you in your situation. Note down topics about which you know little but that are relevant to your work, and calculate if you have further learning needs not met by the article you are reading. If the article is relevant to your practice, record what changes you will make and how you will make the changes. Record how you will impart your new knowledge to others in your practice.

## Educational review

You might find a 'buddy' or work colleague, CPD tutor, or a clinical tutor or clinical supervisor with whom you can have an informal or formal discussion about your performance, job situation and learning needs. You might draw up a learning contract as a result with a timed plan of action.

# Stage 3B: Identify your service needs – how you can find out if there are gaps in your practice

Now focus your attention on the needs of your practice or the PCO. The standards of service delivery should be those that allow you to practise as a competent teacher. You may be competent but be unable to perform or practise to a competent level if the resources available to you are inadequate, or other colleagues have insufficient knowledge or skills to support you. You cannot be expected to take responsibility for ensuring that resources you need to be able to practise in a competent manner are available. However, as a professional you should play a significant role in collecting evidence to make a case for the need for essential resources to your GP colleagues, the practice manager, staff at the trust or PCO or whoever is appropriate.

Some of the methods you might use are described below and include:

- involving learners in giving you feedback about the quality and quantity of your teaching
- monitoring access and availability to teaching – how often are tutorials cancelled due to service needs?
- undertaking a force-field analysis
- assessing the risk of unsupervised learners in the practice
- evaluating the standards of teaching you provide
- comparing the systems in your practice with those required by legislation
- considering your learners' specific needs
- reviewing teamwork and the share of teaching responsibility
- reflecting on whether you are providing quality educational opportunities
- reflecting on whether you are providing cost-effective educational opportunities.

## Involve learners in giving you feedback about the quality and quantity of your teaching

This involvement may occur at three levels:

1  for individual learners about their own needs
2  for learners in general about the range and quality of educational opportunities on offer
3  in planning and organising teaching practice developments.

This process is parallel to 'patient and public involvement', meaning individual involvement as a user, patient or carer, or public involvement that includes the processes of consultation and participation.[17]

Before you involve learners or groups of learners (such as registrars in the vocational training scheme):

- define the purpose
- be realistic about the magnitude of the planned exercise
- select an appropriate method or several methods depending on the target population and your resources

- obtain the commitment of everyone who will be affected by the exercise
- frame the method in accordance with your perspective
- write the protocol.

You might hold focus groups, or invite feedback and help from an established learner group such as a young practitioners' group or higher professional education study group. You could interview learners selected either at random or for their experience of a particular condition or their circumstances.

# Monitor access and availability to teaching – how often are tutorials cancelled due to service needs?

## Access and availability

Do you have regular tutorials with your learners? Is there protected time for teaching that is bleep free or when you are not on call? How many times in, say, a three-month period did all the scheduled teaching sessions actually occur? How prepared are you for teaching – do you sometimes turn up not knowing what the subject is for a tutorial or not having prepared for it? These and other questions are suitable for audit and you or your learner could easily monitor performance.

## Involvement of other team members in teaching

Identify any learning needs here. Have other team members got teaching qualifications or experience? How involved are the nurses in teaching? Could other partners attend a trainers or 'teaching the teachers' course?

# Draw up a force-field analysis

This tool will help you to identify and focus down on the positive and negative forces in your work and to gain an overview of the weighting of these factors. Draw a horizontal or vertical line in the middle of a sheet of paper. Label one side 'positive' and the other side 'negative'. Draw bars to represent individual positive drivers that motivate you on one side of the line, and factors that are demotivating on the other negative side of the line. The thickness and length of the bars should represent the extent of the influence; that is, a short, narrow bar will indicate that the positive or negative factor has a minor influence and a long, wide bar a major effect. See Box 2.5 for an example.

---

**Box 2.5:**  Example of force-field analysis diagram. Satisfaction with current post as a health professional

| Positive factors (driving forces) | Negative factors (restraining forces) |
|---|---|
| career aspirations | long hours of work |
| salary | demands from patients |
| autonomy | |
| satisfaction from caring | job insecurity |
| no uniform | oppressive hierarchy |
| opportunities for professional development | teaching workload |

---

Take an overview of the resulting force-field diagram and consider if you are content with things as they are, or can think of ways to boost the positive side and minimise the negative factors. You can do this part of the exercise on your own, with a peer or a small group in the practice, or with a mentor or someone from outside the practice. The exercise should help you to realise the extent to which a known influence in your life, or in the practice as a whole, is a positive or negative factor. Make a personal or organisational action plan to create the situations and opportunities to boost the positive factors in your life and minimise the bars on the negative side.

## Assess the risk of having learners in the practice

Risk assessment might entail evaluating the risks to the health or wellbeing or competence of yourself, staff and/or patients in your practice or workplace, and deciding on the action needed to minimise or eliminate those risks.[18]

- *A hazard*: something with the potential to cause harm.
- *A risk*: the likelihood of that potential to cause harm being realised.

There are five steps to risk assessment:

1   Look for and list the hazards.
2   Decide who might be harmed and how.
3   Evaluate the risks arising from the hazards and decide whether existing precautions are adequate or more should be done.
4   Record the findings.
5   Review your assessment from time to time and revise it if necessary.

You do not want to spend a lot of time and effort identifying risks or making changes if they do not matter much. When you have identified a risk, consider:

•   is the risk large?
•   does it happen often?
•   is it a significant risk?

Risks may be prevented, avoided, minimised or managed where they cannot be eliminated. You, your colleagues and your staff may need to learn how to do this.

Record significant events where someone has experienced an adverse event or had a near miss – as part of you identifying your service development needs on an ongoing basis. Most significant incidents do not have one cause. Usually there are faults in the system, which are compounded by someone or several people being careless, tired, overworked or ill-informed. Cultivate an atmosphere of openness and discussion without blame so that you can all learn from the significant event. If people think they will be blamed they will hide the incident and no one will be able to prevent it happening again. Look for *all* the causes and try to remedy as many as possible to prevent the situation from arising in the future.

## Evaluate the standards of teaching you provide

Keep your evaluation as simple as possible. Avoid wasting resources on unnecessarily bureaucratic evaluation. Design the evaluation so that you:

•   specify the event (e.g. a teaching programme) to be evaluated – define broad issues, set priorities against strategic goals, time and resources, seek agreement on the nature and scope of the task
•   describe the expected impact of the programme or activity and who will be affected
•   define the criteria of success – these might relate to structure, process or outcome
•   identify the information required to demonstrate the achievements of the programme or activity. The record might include: learner feedback, observing behaviour, data from existing records, prospective recording by

the learners of the programme or measurement of change in behaviour following the teaching
* determine the time frame for the evaluation
* specify who collects the data for all stages in the delivery of the programme or activity, and the respective deadlines
* review and refine the objectives of the programme or activity and check that they are appropriate for the outcomes and impact you expect.

## What to evaluate?

You could:

* adopt any, or all, of the six aspects of the health service's performance assessment framework (*see* Box 2.6)
* agree milestones and goals at stages in your programme
* evaluate the extent to which you achieve the outcome(s) starting with an objective. Alternatively, you might evaluate how conducive is the context of the programme, or activity, to achieving the anticipated outcomes
* undertake regular audits of aspects of the structure, process and outcome of a service or project to see if you have achieved what you expected when you established the criteria and standards of the audit programme
* evaluate the various components of a new system or programme: the activities, personnel involved, provision of services, organisational structure, precise goals and interventions.

---

**Box 2.6:**   The six aspects of the NHS performance assessment framework
1   Health improvement
2   Fair access
3   Effective delivery
4   Efficiency
5   Patient/carer (learner) experience
6   Health outcomes

---

Look at your learning or teaching practice development needs by maintaining appropriate records to enable you to:

* look at trends and patterns of learner feedback
* audit what you are doing
* provide the information on which to base decisions on commissioning and management
* support epidemiology and research as well as teaching activities.

# Compare the systems in your practice with those required by legislation

Legislation changes quite frequently and the criteria for a training practice, for example, are modified from time to time. As an employer, a GP needs to keep abreast of the legislation or ensure that the practice manager does so. You could start by comparing the systems in your practice with those required by the Disability Discrimination Act (1995) and health and safety legislation. GPs are designated employers of registrars and liable under equal opportunities legislation as well.

# Consider your learners' specific needs

What do you know about the learners you are responsible for? What are their circumstances and backgrounds? What is their employment background and experience? There is no need for you to pry into their private life but a certain awareness of conflicting obligations, such as childcare, is useful. Awareness of where they have worked and positions they have held before helps you tailor your teaching to their requirements.

Have you paid attention to their learning styles? Are you comfortable teaching in different styles to match differing learners' needs?

What postgraduate or other exams are they preparing for? How do they study? All these inquiries can be looked at and the outcomes included as evidence that you are aware of learner difference.

# Review teamwork

You can measure how effective the team is – evaluate whether the team has:[19]

- clear goals and objectives
- accountability and authority
- individual roles for members
- shared tasks
- regular internal formal and informal communication
- full participation by members
- confrontation of conflict
- feedback to individuals
- feedback about team performance
- outside recognition
- two-way external communication
- team rewards.

Would you know if there were others in your team who wanted to share the teaching? Are there some who would rather opt out?

# Reflect on whether you are providing quality educational opportunities

Quality may be subdivided into eight components: equity, access, acceptability and responsiveness, appropriateness, communication, continuity, effectiveness and efficiency.[20]

You might use the matrix in Box 2.7 as a way of ordering your approach to auditing a particular topic with the eight aspects of quality on the vertical axis and structure, process and outcome on the horizontal axis.[21] In this way you can generate up to 24 aspects of a particular topic.

---

**Box 2.7:**   Matrix for assessing the quality of educational provision

You might like to look at the structure, process or outcome of video recording consultations with learners, for example:

|                                   | Structure              | Process                    | Outcome                   |
| --------------------------------- | ---------------------- | -------------------------- | ------------------------- |
| Equity                            |                        |                            |                           |
| Access                            |                        |                            |                           |
| Acceptability and responsiveness  |                        |                            |                           |
| Appropriateness                   |                        |                            |                           |
| Communication                     | Consent forms in place | Instructions for patients  | Consultation technique    |
| Continuity                        |                        |                            |                           |
| Effectiveness                     |                        |                            |                           |
| Efficiency                        |                        |                            |                           |

---

Look for service development needs reflecting why learners receive a poor quality of service such as:

- inadequately trained staff or staff with poor levels of competence
- lack of confidentiality
- educational supervisors not being contactable in an emergency or being ineffective
- teaching being unavailable due to poor management of resources or services
- insufficient numbers of available staff for the workload.

Many of these items will need action as a team, but for some of them, it may be your responsibility to ensure that adequate standards are met.

# Reflect on whether you are providing cost-effective healthcare or education

Cost-effectiveness is not synonymous with 'cheap'. A cost-effective intervention is one which gives a better or equivalent benefit from the intervention in question for lower or equivalent cost, or where the relative improvement in outcome is higher than the relative difference in cost. In other words being cost-effective means having the best outcomes for the least input. Using the term 'cost-effective' implies that you have considered potential alternatives.

Do the arrangements for teaching in your team represent good value for money? Is it cost-effective for you to take time out to teach?

An economic evaluation is a comparative analysis of two or more alternatives in terms of their costs and consequences. There are four different types as shown in Box 2.8.

---

**Box 2.8:**   The four types of economic evaluation

1   *Cost-effectiveness analysis* is used to compare the effectiveness of two interventions with the same objectives.
2   *Cost minimisation* compares the costs of alternative strategies that have identical educational outcomes.
3   *Cost–utility analysis* enables the effects of alternative interventions to be measured against an outcome measure such as numbers of trainees passing summative assessment.
4   *Cost–benefit analysis* is a technique designed to determine the feasibility of a project, plan, or strategy by quantifying its costs and benefits. It is often difficult to determine these accurately in relation to education.

---

While educational evaluation is unavoidable, it cannot be objective. You will probably have learning needs around what subjective method is best to use.[22]

Efficiency is sometimes confused with effectiveness. Being efficient means obtaining the most quality from the least expenditure, or the required level of quality for the least expenditure. To measure efficiency you need to make a judgement about the level of quality of the 'purchase' and be able to relate it to 'price'. 'Price' alone does not measure efficiency. Quality is the indicator used in combination with price to assess if something is more efficient. So, cost-effectiveness is a measure of efficiency and suggests that costs have been related to effectiveness.

Consider if you have service development needs. Discuss whether:

- the current skill mix in your team is appropriate
- more cost-effective alternative types of delivery of education are available
- sufficient staff training exists for those taking on new roles and responsibilities.

# Set priorities: how you match what's needed with what's possible

You and your colleagues will have been able to make a wish list after following the previous Stages 3A and 3B undertaking a variety of needs assessments. Group and summarise your learning and service development needs from the exercises you have carried out. Grade them according to the priority you set. You may put one at a higher priority because it fits in with learning needs established from another section, or put another lower because it does not fit in with other activities that you will put into your learning plan for the next 12 months. If you have identified a learning need by several different methods of assessment then it will have a higher priority than something only identified once in your PDP. Collect information from all the team, the patients, users and carers to feed back before you make a decision on how to progress. Remember to take external influences into account such as the National Service Frameworks, National Institute for Clinical Excellence (NICE) guidance, governmental priorities, priorities of your PCO, the content of the Local Delivery Plan, etc. Try to gain a balance between the teaching and clinical components of your everyday work.

Select those topics that are tied into your developmental priorities, have clear aims and objectives and are achievable within your time and resource constraints. When ranking topics for learning or action in order of priority (Stage 4) consider whether:

- the project aims and objectives are clearly defined
- the topic is important:
  - for the population served (e.g. the size of the problem and/or its severity)
  - for the skills, knowledge or attitudes of the individual or team
- it is feasible
- it is affordable
- it will make enough difference
- it fits in with other priorities.

You will still have more ideas than can possibly be implemented. Remember the highest priority – the health service is for patients that use it or who will do so in the future.

# References

1  Medical Professionalism Project (2002) Medical professionalism in the new millennium: a physicians' charter. *Lancet.* **359**: 520–2.

2  Eraut M and du Boulay B (2000) *Developing the Attributes of Medical Professional Judgement and Competence.* University of Sussex, Sussex. Reproduced at http://www.cogs.susx.ac.uk/users/bend/doh.

3  Fraser SW and Greenhalgh T (2001) Coping with complexity: educating for capability. *British Medical Journal.* **323**: 799–802.

4  General Medical Council (2001) *Good Medical Practice.* General Medical Council, London.

5  Pendleton D, Schofield T, Tate P and Havelock P (2003) *The New Consultation, Developing Doctor–Patient Communication.* Oxford University Press, Oxford.

6  King J (2002) Career focus: 360° appraisal. *British Medical Journal.* **324**: S195.

7  Royal College of General Practitioners/General Practitioners' Committee (2002) *Good Medical Practice for General Practitioners.* Royal College of General Practitioners, London.

8  Irvine D and Irvine S (eds) (1991) *Making Sense of Audit.* Radcliffe Medical Press, Oxford.

9  Toon P, Greenhalgh T, Rigby M *et al.* (2002) *The Human Face of Medicine.* Two CD ROMs in the APOLLO (Advancing Professional Practice through Online Learning Opportunities) series. BMJ Publishing Group, London. Free sample available at www.apollobmj.com.

10  www.eguidelines.co.uk.

11  www.doctors.net.uk.

12  www.npcrdc.man.ac.uk.

13  http://latis.ex.ac.uk/cfep/index.htm.

14  Department of Health (2003) EPP Update newsletter. Department of Health, London. See Expert Patient Programme on www.ohn.gov.uk/ohn/people/expert.htm.

15  Department of Health (2003) *The NHS Knowledge and Skills Framework (NHS KSF) and Development Review Guidance – working draft.* Version 6. Department of Health, London.

16  Department of Health (2003) *Job Evaluation Handbook.* Version 1. Department of Health, London.

17  Chambers R, Drinkwater C and Boath E (2003) *Involving Patients and the Public: how to do it better* (2e). Radcliffe Medical Press, Oxford.

18  Mohanna K and Chambers R (2000) *Risk Matters in Healthcare.* Radcliffe Medical Press, Oxford.

19 Hart E and Fletcher J (1999) Learning how to change: a selective analysis of literature and experience of how teams learn and organisations change. *Journal of Interprofessional Care.* **13 (1)**: 53–63.

20 Maxwell RJ (1984) Quality assessment in health. *British Medical Journal.* **288**: 1470–2.

21 Firth-Cozens J (1993) *Audit in Mental Health Services.* Lawrence Erlbaum Associates, Hove.

22 McCulloch D (2003) *Valuing Health in Practice.* Ashgate Publishing Ltd, Aldershot.

# 3

## Demonstrating common components of good quality healthcare

In looking at the quality of teaching you provide and demonstrating your standards of service delivery and outcomes of learning, you should find that obtaining informed consent from patients to be involved in teaching, maintaining confidentiality while teaching, and handling complaints from patients involved in teaching scenarios are part of the fabric of good quality care.

These three aspects are included in this chapter to introduce the concept of the evidence cycle. The examples given here are not specific to your teaching role, they can be adapted and modified as need be. But they are presented here in generic form as a starting point.

We have set out the chapter with key information about consent followed by some example cycles of the stages of evidence (*see* Figure 1.1 on page 6). The two other sections on confidentiality and complaints follow, laid out in similar ways. Read through the cycles of evidence to become familiar with the approach to gathering and documenting evidence of your learning, competence, performance or standards of service delivery. Then either adopt one of the examples or adapt it to your own teaching practice. Alternatively, read on to one or more of the 'aspects of education' chapters that follow and look at these three components in a different context such as in developing self-directed learners or giving feedback.

## Consent

### Key points

Information given to a health professional remains the property of the patient. In most circumstances, consent is assumed for the necessary sharing of information with other professionals involved with the care of the patient for that episode of care. Usually consent is also assumed for essential sharing of information for continuing care. Beyond this, informed consent must be obtained. Patients attend for healthcare in the belief that the personal information that they supply, or which is found out about them during investigation or treatment, will be confidential.

Exceptions to the above[1] are:

- if the patient consents
- if it is in the patient's own interest that information should be disclosed, but it is either impossible to seek the patient's consent or
- it is medically undesirable in the patient's own interest, to seek the patient's consent
- if the law requires (and does not merely permit) the health professional to disclose the information
- if the health professional has an overriding duty to society to disclose the information
- if the health professional agrees with a governmental agency that disclosure is necessary to safeguard national security
- if the disclosure is necessary to prevent a serious risk to public health
- in certain circumstances, for the purposes of medical research.

> Health professionals must be able to justify their decision to disclose information without consent. If they are in any doubt, they should consult their professional bodies and colleagues.

Consent is only valid if the patient fully understands the nature and consequences of disclosure – they must be able to give their consent, receive enough information to enable them to make a decision and be acting under their own free will and not persuaded by the strong influence of another person. If consent is given, the health worker is responsible for limiting the disclosure to that information for which informed consent has been obtained. The development of modern information technology and the increasing amount of multidisciplinary teamwork in patient care make confidentiality difficult to uphold.

You may need to give information about a patient to a relative or carer. Normally the consent of the patient should be obtained. Sometimes, the clinical condition of the patient may prevent informed consent being obtained (e.g. they are unconscious or have a severe illness). It is important to recognise that relatives or carers do *not* have any right to information about the patient. Disclosure without consent may be justified when third parties are exposed to a risk so serious that it outweighs the patient's privacy. An example would be if a patient declines to allow you to disclose information about their health and continues to drive against medical advice when unfit to do so.

Local research ethics committees and the research governance framework ensure best practice in the giving of informed consent by patients in research studies.

As health professionals, we often assume implied consent. The general public and patients are generally ignorant of the extent to which information about them is passed around the NHS. When teaching at both undergraduate and postgraduate levels, in examinations and assessments and in research we may incorrectly assume patients imply their consent. Consent is also implied for health service accounting, central monitoring of referrals, in disease registers, for audit and in facilitating joint working between team members. The NHS is still engaged in a debate about what data can legitimately be shared without patients' explicit consent. Although written consent is usually obtained for supplying information to insurance companies or for legal reports, patients are often unaware of the type of information being supplied and have not given 'informed consent'. Guidelines published jointly by the British Medical Association (BMA) and the Association of British Insurers clarify that doctors are not required to release all aspects of a patient's medical history but need only submit (with the patient's consent) information that is relevant.[2]

The GMC's booklet *Seeking Patients' Consent: the ethical considerations* explores issues of consent in more depth and advises that:

> the amount of information you give each patient will vary according to factors such as the nature of the condition, the complexity of the treatment, the risks associated with the treatment or procedure and the patient's own wishes ... you should be careful about relying on a patient's apparent compliance with a procedure as a form of consent.[3]

# Collecting data to demonstrate your learning, competence, performance and standards of service delivery: consent

## Example cycle of evidence 3.1

- Focus: informed consent
- Other relevant focus: relationships with patients

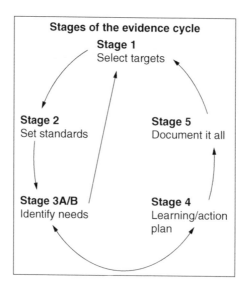

Stages of the evidence cycle

Stage 1
Select targets

Stage 2
Set standards

Stage 5
Document it all

Stage 3A/B
Identify needs

Stage 4
Learning/action plan

---

**Box 3.1:** Case study

While you have a colleague who has just started in special interest training with you, Mrs Bowed comes to see you about her contraception. You sketch out the alternatives that are open to her as a 35-year-old smoker. It transpires that she has had unprotected sexual intercourse four days previously and is at risk of pregnancy. You advise that she should have an intrauterine device (IUD) fitted straightaway, as this will provide emergency contraception and long-term contraception. 'I might as well – you know best' she says passively, with a long sigh. Further discussion reveals that she felt pressured to have a termination of pregnancy by her mother when a teenager, with which the doctors colluded. Since then, she's never taken any real decisions about her health or contraception, having had a domineering husband who has recently left her.

> This is just an example. Keep your task simple. You could choose three or four cycles of evidence to demonstrate your competence each year.

## Stage 1: Select your aspirations for good practice

The excellent health professional:

- obtains informed consent to treatment
- treats patients politely and with consideration.

## Stage 2: Set the standards for your outcomes

Outcomes might include:

- a tutorial plan
- mastery of a new skill as a teacher
- a teaching strategy that is implemented
- learner feedback
- evaluation of teaching programmes.

- A completed audit that shows that you, or all clinicians in the team, consistently obtain women's informed consent to treatment or other clinical management.
- Devise, apply and act on appropriate patient survey tool that ascertains patients' views about their treatment by yourself, others in the practice or directorate team, e.g. establishing views as to whether you treat patients politely and with consideration.
- You might choose to focus on referral for termination of pregnancy, or consent for contraception such as an injection, the fitting of an IUD or implant, or for investigations such as taking vaginal swabs.

## Stage 3A: Identify your learning needs

- Review the consent and communication issues in a complaint or expression of discontent made by a patient to any member of the practice or ward team.
- Reflect on whether you follow best practice in obtaining and recording consent to treatment or procedures.

## Stage 3B: Identify your service needs

> Any of the needs assessment exercises in 3A may also reveal service needs.

- Compare the consent policy in your practice or directorate against recommended best practice or another consent policy and reflect on the differences.
- Audit the case notes to determine whether doctors and nurses recorded the discussion of parental knowledge and consent to treatment with contraception in consultations with under-16 year olds.
- Undertake a targeted teenage patient survey. You might look at teenagers who have consulted you and others at the surgery. Alternatively, you might learn more from a survey of teenagers at a local youth centre, as this would include non-users of NHS services. You could ask about any aspect of teenage health, such as their experiences of informed consent, or how treatment options have been explained, or their experience of consultations with local GPs or nurses, relating to politeness and consideration.

## Stage 4: Make and carry out a learning and action plan

- Identify the issues from the learning and service needs assessment exercises in Stages 3A and 3B, e.g. comparing your own consent policy with others.
- Set up a workshop on communication skills highlighting politeness and consideration, and ability to gain informed consent, e.g. by video recording and reflection/feedback with various types of patients including teenagers.
- Arrange and attend a facilitated meeting with a group of women to discuss their experiences of consulting health professionals, to gain their opinions about access, the welcome, and general attitudes in the surgery e.g. organised by the patient participation group.

## Stage 5: Document your learning, competence, performance and standards of service delivery

- Make notes of the review of the complaint or adverse comments and subsequent plan to minimise likelihood of re-occurrence.
- Repeat the initial learning or service needs assessments, e.g. re-audit and repeat the patient survey.
- Audit that the consent policy is applied consistently by all clinical members of the practice team, e.g. from case notes, patient feedback, self-report. You might find that consent is reported as being obtained but not recorded in the patients' records. This would imply that a change in recording practice is required and produce future new learning needs!

---

**Box 3.2:**   Case study continued

You help Mrs Bowed to understand the risk and consequences of pregnancy and the urgency of action she needs to take if she wishes to receive emergency contraception. You talk through the advantages and disadvantages of the fitting of an IUD and its use as long-term contraception. You suggest an assertiveness course run by the local further education college she might like to consider. You arrange for her to have the IUD fitted later the same day when she has had an opportunity to reflect about what she wants to do and has given informed consent to the fitting. You discuss the pitfalls of over-compliant behaviour with your colleague who is in training with you.

---

# Example cycle of evidence 3.2

- Focus: informed consent
- Other relevant focus: research

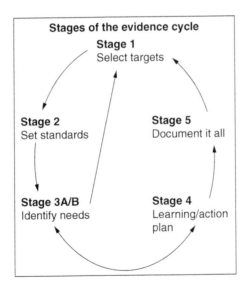

**Stages of the evidence cycle**

Stage 1
Select targets

Stage 2
Set standards

Stage 5
Document it all

Stage 3A/B
Identify needs

Stage 4
Learning/action
plan

**Box 3.3:**   Case study

You agree to undertake a survey to find out if patients are satisfied with your services. The practice manager will organise it, but you are nominated to lead the work. You decide to focus on teenagers as a group as the adolescent drop-in clinic you set up two years ago with the school health service is not being used as much as it once was. You are not sure how to survey the teenagers. You think they are unlikely to answer questionnaires sent through the post and think you will interview teenagers about their satisfaction with the clinic. You intend to employ one of your own teenage children to interview some who have never come to the clinic, by selecting their names from your patient list, as well as some teenagers who have attended. You're not sure if you are getting into research territory or if it is okay to claim you are auditing your services.

This is just an example. Keep your task simple. You could choose three or four cycles of evidence to demonstrate your competence each year.

## Stage 1: Select your aspirations for good practice

The excellent health professional:

- protects patients' rights and makes sure that they are not disadvantaged by taking part in research
- gives patients the information they need about their problem in a way they can understand as a basis for informed consent.

## Stage 2: Set the standards for your outcomes

Outcomes might include:

- a tutorial plan
- mastery of a new skill as a teacher
- a teaching strategy that is implemented
- learner feedback
- evaluation of teaching programmes.

- Informed consent policy of practice covers patients' participation in audit and research as well as consent to clinical treatment.
- You should be able to describe the difference between audit of clinical management and service provision and research.

## Stage 3A: Identify your learning needs

- Read through the frequently asked questions and answers on the Department of Health website relating to research governance.[4] Consider whether you are able to answer the questions before reading the answers.
- Describe an audit plan of the adolescent clinic that involves obtaining young people's views of standards of services by interviewing them. Submit the plan to the chair of the local research ethics committee to check that he/she agrees that the audit proposal does not fall within the definition of research and to approve the patient literature and the process inviting informed consent to take part.

## Stage 3B: Identify your service needs

Any of the needs assessment exercises in 3A may also reveal service needs.

- Draw up an information leaflet for young people about the audit of adolescent clinic services that you intend to carry out. Ask others to critique the leaflet – young people for its readability and clarity, a research colleague for the extent to which it conforms to best practice for informed consent. Use the information leaflet so that they can give informed consent to the interview to obtain their views and audio recording of the interview.
- Ask a colleague to peer review the extent to which advice and information you give to teenagers during a consultation is accurate. The teenager would need to have given prior, written informed consent for the peer review (and audio recording if used).

## Stage 4: Make and carry out a learning and action plan

- Obtain and read documents about research governance from the Department of Health's website or from your PCO – as in section 3A, first point.
- Study the application form for the ethical approval of a research study.
- Understand the limits to obtaining patients' views as part of audit of clinical and service management by reading up on informed consent. Read the GMC's booklet: *Seeking Patients' Consent: the ethical considerations.*[3] Look

at whether you are explaining the details of the diagnosis or prognosis, giving an explanation of likely benefits and side-effects, explaining whether a proposed treatment is experimental and whether a doctor in training will be involved.

- Ask for a short tutorial from your local clinical governance lead about good practice in obtaining patients' views through audit, research and patient involvement activities – including good practice in informed consent.

## Stage 5: Document your learning, competence, performance and standards of service delivery

- Make a comparison of your own practice with the answers to the frequently asked questions on the Department of Health website relating to research governance.[4]
- File a response letter from the chair of the local research ethics committee about the audit proposal.
- Keep the subsequent revised audit plan to ensure that work does not fall within the definition of research.
- Keep the revised patients' informed consent leaflet, following the critique.
- Repeat the peer review by the same, or another, colleague of the extent to which advice and information you give to teenagers during consultations is accurate.

---

**Box 3.4:** Case study continued

The chair of the research ethics committee advises you that your plan should be classed as research rather than audit as it involves contact with patients outside their usual NHS care. He explains about the risks of using untrained interviewers such as your own children and the need to fully inform those teenagers you are inviting to be interviewed about the survey and that their refusal will not prejudice their medical care. He advises you to send an application form for formal approval to the ethics committee and to contact the research lead in your PCO in line with the research governance framework if you wish to continue to develop a research project. You revise your plans as the scale of the work required is becoming out of all proportion.

---

# Example cycle of evidence 3.3

- Focus: informed consent
- Other relevant focus: working with colleagues

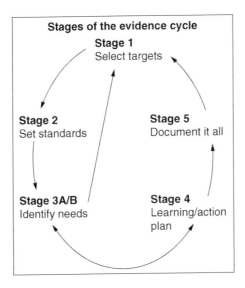

**Stages of the evidence cycle**

**Stage 1**
Select targets

**Stage 2**
Set standards

**Stage 5**
Document it all

**Stage 3A/B**
Identify needs

**Stage 4**
Learning/action
plan

---

**Box 3.5:**   Case study

Miss Young comes with her carer to see you. The carer explains that the new manager of the unit for people with learning disabilities, in which Miss Young lives, wants Miss Young to have a cervical smear and mammography. Although Miss Young is 52 years old she has had neither screening test. You wonder how to proceed, as Miss Young does not seem to have any say in this.

This is just an example. Keep your task simple. You could choose three or four cycles of evidence to demonstrate your competence each year.

## Stage 1: Select your aspirations for good practice

The excellent health professional:

- acts in the best interests of patients when making referrals and providing or arranging treatment or care, acting with patients' informed consent
- makes sure that others understand their professional status and speciality, what roles and responsibilities they have and who is responsible for each aspect of the patient's care.

## Stage 2: Set the standards for your outcomes

Outcomes might include:

- a tutorial plan
- mastery of a new skill as a teacher
- a teaching strategy that is implemented
- learner feedback
- evaluation of teaching programmes.

- Publish a practice or hospital policy on informed consent for patients with mental health problems and learning disabilities, including dementia.

## Stage 3A: Identify your learning needs

- Analyse a significant event, e.g. you referred Miss Young for mammography and she refuses to co-operate in the X-ray department resulting in telephoned protest from the radiographer.
- Self-assessment – you are aware that you do not know how to proceed (e.g. in the consultation in the case study). You do not know how much you can rely on the carer having already gained Miss Young's informed consent or the extent to which you can take Miss Young's acquiescence for 'consent'.
- Read up and reflect on the association between competency or capacity to be well informed and the degree of previous education and the inability of some individuals to provide informed consent if they have educational, social and cultural reasons that limit their understanding of complex issues.

## Stage 3B: Identify your service needs

Any of the needs assessment exercises in 3A may also reveal service needs.

- Carry out a review of case notes of women aged 20–65 years old with learning disabilities to determine the numbers who have had cervical smears, mammograms, immunisations, etc.
- Arrange a focus group discussion with people with learning disabilities and their carers (or other target group such as people with dementia and their carers) to discuss the appropriateness of the patient's consent process for all clinical interventions including cervical cytology and mammography.

## Stage 4: Make and carry out a learning and action plan

- Ask advice from MENCAP about the approach they recommend for obtaining informed consent from 'vulnerable' groups of people, how to explain clinical management and pursue clinical interventions, together with any associated useful literature.
- Read up on informed consent.
- Revise the practice informed consent policy to include specific groups of 'vulnerable' people such as those with learning disabilities or mental ill-health problems.

## Stage 5: Document your learning, competence, performance and standards of service delivery

- Run a quiz for members of the practice team at an in-house educational event with four hypothetical cases. Compare the answers with best practice according to MENCAP[5] and other professional literature.
- Include the revised practice policy on informed consent.
- Audit the consistent application of the revised practice informed consent policy with consecutive cases, e.g. search on people coded as having learning disability on computer. Look to see what interventions have been undertaken and whether informed consent has been recorded in the notes.
- Use specimen consent forms that have been piloted, revised and audited.

---

**Box 3.6:**   Case study continued

Miss Young returns for a follow-up appointment, having been left at the last surgery appointment to think about having a cervical smear and with a referral for mammography. She has told her carer that she has had some bleeding from down below so a pelvic examination and smear are warranted clinically. You take plenty of time to explain how you will do the pelvic examination and smear, Miss Young agrees and all goes well.

---

# Confidentiality

## Key points

You should have appropriate confidentiality safeguards in place in the practice to prevent inadvertent disclosure of personal and sensitive information about patients. Tell people, especially the young, about their right to confidential medical treatment and reinforce your conversation with posters and leaflets. People with non-prescription drug-related problems who seek help from substance abuse clinics, or those with sexually transmitted infections who attend genitourinary medicine clinics, often do not want their GP to be told because they do not believe that the information will be kept confidential. Fears about confidentiality are the commonest reason young people give for not attending their GP for contraceptive treatment.[6]

Young people under the age of 16 years have the same rights to confidentiality as other patients. The younger the person, the greater care is needed to assess the level of understanding to ensure that he or she understands the consequences of any proposed action. If a young person fulfils the conditions given in Box 3.7, he or she is regarded as being competent to make his or her own decisions.

---

**Box 3.7:**   The Fraser Guidelines[7]

The guidelines were drawn up after Lord Fraser stated in 1985 that a doctor could give contraceptive advice or treatment to a person under 16 years old without parental consent, providing that the doctor is satisfied that:

- the young person will understand the advice
- the young person cannot be persuaded to tell their parents or allow the doctor to tell them that they are seeking contraceptive advice
- the young person is likely to begin or continue having unprotected sex with or without contraceptive treatment
- the young person's physical or mental health is likely to suffer unless they receive contraceptive advice or treatment
- it is in the young person's best interest to receive contraceptive advice or treatment.

The Fraser Guidelines apply to health professionals in England and Wales. In Scotland, the Age of Legal Capacity (Scotland) Act 1991 gives similar powers of consent to those under 16 years of age.

In Northern Ireland, although separate legislation applies, the then Department of Health and Social Services Northern Ireland stated that there was no reason to suppose that the House of Lords' decision would not be followed by the Northern Ireland Courts.

---

Occasionally you may feel that you have a moral obligation to divulge confidential information. Whenever possible you should seek to persuade the patient to give consent to the disclosure. Seek advice from your professional organisations in circumstances where others are at danger (e.g. risk of harm, or rape or sexual abuse), or where a serious crime has been committed. Health professionals should satisfy themselves that sufficient authority has been obtained (e.g. a certificate from the Attorney General or Lord Advocate) and consult professional organisations before disclosing information without a patient's consent.

---

**Box 3.8:**   The Caldicott Committee Report

The Caldicott Committee Report described principles of good practice to safeguard confidentiality when information is being used for non-clinical purposes:[8]

- justify the purpose
- do not use patient-identifiable information unless it is absolutely necessary
- use the minimum necessary patient-identifiable information
- access to patient-identifiable information should be on a strict need-to-know basis
- everyone with access to patient-identifiable information should be aware of his or her responsibilities.

---

Interpreters should be used wherever possible to avoid the use of friends or relatives. They should be trained in the requirements of confidentiality.

Patients are entitled to access data held about them. Exceptions to this right are:

- the patient failed to make the request in accordance with the Data Protection Act 1998
- if acceding to the request would result in disclosure of information about somebody else without their consent
- when giving medical information may cause serious harm to the mental or physical health of the patient (a rare occurrence).

You need to incorporate systems for ensuring that paper and computer security are maintained. Systems for monitoring and upgrading security systems should be in place and you should check regularly that confidentiality is not being breached if changes are made.

# Collecting data to demonstrate your learning, competence, performance and standards of service delivery: confidentiality

## Example cycle of evidence 3.4

- Focus: confidentiality
- Other relevant focus: teaching and training

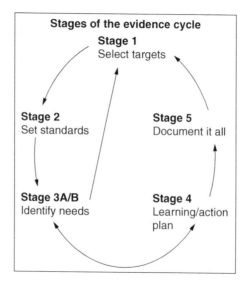

**Stages of the evidence cycle**

**Stage 1**
Select targets

**Stage 2**
Set standards

**Stage 3A/B**
Identify needs

**Stage 4**
Learning/action plan

**Stage 5**
Document it all

---

**Box 3.9:**   Case study

It is the first time you have had students placed with you and you want to teach two of them about the importance of making sure that young people under-stand the practice or hospital code on confidentiality while they are on their placement with you.

---

This is just an example. Keep your task simple. You could choose three or four cycles of evidence to demonstrate your competence each year.

## Stage 1: Select your aspirations for good practice

The excellent health professional:

- maintains the confidentiality of patient-specific information
- ensures that patients are not put at risk when seeing students or doctors in training.

## Stage 2: Set the standards for your outcomes

Outcomes might include:

- a tutorial plan
- mastery of a new skill as a teacher
- a teaching strategy that is implemented
- learner feedback
- evaluation of teaching programmes.

- Ensure that all members of the practice team including you, new members of staff and students or doctors in training are familiar with guidelines for confidentiality.

## Stage 3A: Identify your learning needs

- Assess your knowledge about the limits of confidentiality, e.g. for providing under-16 year olds with contraception or referring them for termination of pregnancy or other surgical intervention.
- Ask an expert tutor's opinion about the particular method of teaching you plan to use for an in-house training session on maintaining confidentiality for teenagers of different ages that will best convey main messages and lead to changes where necessary.

## Stage 3B: Identify your service needs

Any of the needs assessment exercises in 3A may also reveal service needs.

- Compare the practice or hospital protocol for confidentiality with the guidelines in the *Confidentiality and Young People* toolkit.[6]
- Review the intended induction programme for new members of staff, students on placement and doctors in training, to assess the extent to which knowledge of confidentiality features and is addressed.

*Stage 4: Make and carry out a learning and action plan*

- Find out from the local educational tutor how to undertake learning needs assessments of others from different disciplines with different levels of responsibilities in respect of confidentiality.
- Prepare for and run an interactive teaching session on confidentiality for patients of all age groups with special focus on teenagers. You might invite the whole practice team, including students, family planning or school nurses, local pharmacists, GP registrars, etc. You could use the *Confidentiality and Young People* toolkit for promoting discussion with the practice team at the session.[6]

*Stage 5: Document your learning, competence, performance and standards of service delivery*

- Run a quiz completed by those attending the teaching session before and after training about confidentiality.
- Create an incident record kept by the team of any reported or perceived breaches of confidentiality by anyone working in, or associated with, the practice.
- Ensure the existence of personal learning plans based on learning needs assessments for new staff or doctors in training by the end of their induction period.
- Revise the practice or hospital protocol in line with the *Confidentiality and Young People* toolkit.[6]

---

**Box 3.10:**   Case study continued

Other staff colleagues join your teaching session with the students using the video from the *Confidentiality and Young People* toolkit.[6] All get full marks in the quiz after watching the video.

---

# Learning from complaints

## Key points

There is learning to be had from every complaint. The GMC received a record 5539 complaints in 2002, 4% more than in 2001; of these, 72 resulted in a doctor being banned or suspended.[9] Even if the complaint is trivial or undeserved, it implies a lack of communication. Table 3.1 describes the nature of claims against GPs reported in a study of 1000 consecutive clinical cases. There are a myriad of associated reasons for the claims. Many of the clinical events will reveal failings in the practice systems and processes and in the practice of the health professional – such as communication, diagnostic skills, etc.

**Table 3.1:**   The nature of 1000 claims against GPs handled by the Medical Protection Society[10]

| Claim by patient | Number of claims |
|---|---|
| Problems of diagnosis (delayed or missed) | 631 |
| Prescribing errors | 193 |
| Malignant neoplasms (some of the problems of diagnosis) | 140 |
|    Cancer of the breast (lumpiness often falsely diagnosed as benign) | 20 |
|    Cancer of the cervix (often abnormalities filed away and not acted upon) | 14 |
|    Cancer of the digestive organs (cancer of the colon most frequent with misdiagnosed symptoms) | 21 |
| Diabetes (8 deaths) primary failure to diagnose (19 delays in diagnosis) (9 delays in referral of patient resulting in amputation) | 40 |
| Myocardial infarction 27 deaths (8 undiagnosed, 7 diagnosed as dyspepsia, 3 diagnosed as congestive cardiac failure, 3 as muscular origin, 2 as chest infection) | 34 |
| Prescribing | |
|    Steroids (e.g. osteoporotic collapse) | 40 |
|    Antibiotic allergy | 8 |
|    Phenothiazines (extrapyramidal symptoms) | 10 |
|    Hormone replacement therapy | 9 |
|    Oral contraception | 9 |
|    Warfarin (interactions e.g. resulting in cerebral haemorrhage) | 5 |

# Collecting data to demonstrate your learning, competence, performance and standards of service delivery: complaints

## Example cycle of evidence 3.5

- Focus: complaints
- Other relevant focus of evidence: working with colleagues

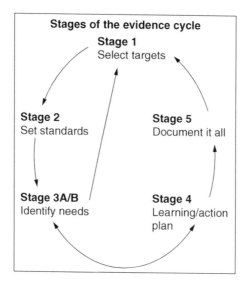

Stages of the evidence cycle

Stage 1
Select targets

Stage 2
Set standards

Stage 5
Document it all

Stage 3A/B
Identify needs

Stage 4
Learning/action plan

---

**Box 3.11:** Case study

Your practice has received a patient complaint about a GP locum failing to diagnose a patient's bowel cancer on the first occasion they consulted. This has prompted you all as a practice team to review the way that your complaints system functions.

---

This is just an example. Keep your task simple. You could choose three or four cycles of evidence to demonstrate your competence each year.

## Stage 1: Select your aspirations for good practice

The excellent health professional:

- apologises appropriately when things go wrong, and has an adequate complaints procedure in place.

## Stage 2: Set the standards for your outcomes

Outcomes might include:

- a tutorial plan
- mastery of a new skill as a teacher
- a teaching strategy that is implemented
- learner feedback
- evaluation of teaching programmes.

- Understand and establish effective processes for preventing and managing complaints from patients in the practice.

## Stage 3A: Identify your learning needs

- Examine as a significant event one or more complaints, e.g. where the practice has not advised a patient correctly about the complaints process.
- Compare the actual care of a patient against an acceptable standard of care for a range of clinical conditions as ongoing review for a clinical area that has been the subject of a complaint (e.g. bowel cancer in case study). You could use peer review by asking respected colleagues or compare your practice against a published standard such as a guideline by a responsible body of professional opinion.

## Stage 3B: Identify your service needs

Any of the needs assessment exercises in 3A may also reveal service needs.

- Audit patient complaints in the preceding 12 months: the number, the outcomes and how the complaint system is advertised, etc.
- Audit the extent to which doctors and nurses are following practice-agreed protocols. This is about being proactive about preventing or minimising the likelihood of the source of the complaint recurring.

- Audit vulnerable areas. Look back at the analysis of complaints to identify useful areas for focusing learning, e.g. a review of the prescribing of steroids.
- Review the way that the qualifications of locums are checked and that they are made aware of the practice protocols.

## Stage 4: Make and carry out a learning and action plan

- Ask your PCO to look at the practice complaints system and feed back how it can be improved (if at all).
- Arrange a tutorial between the practice manager and others in the team about preventing and managing complaints, or use one of the risk management packages produced by medical defence organisations.[11,12]
- Read up on how to undertake significant event analysis including how to share the information with the practice team and respond as a practice team.

## Stage 5: Document your learning, competence, performance and standards of service delivery

- Collect evidence of clinical competence to guard against a complaint.
- Develop a protocol of the patient complaint process against which consecutive complaints can be audited in another 12 months' time.
- Document guidance about physical examinations including that the reason for any examination should be communicated clearly, that a chaperone should be offered for any internal or breast examination, and the comfort and privacy of the patient should always be kept in mind to avoid potential complaints.
- Make sure a file containing practice protocols is available for easy reference on the desktop of the computer.

---

**Box 3.12:**   Case study continued

You are invited by your PCO to take a lead in advising GPs in other practices about the handling of complaints because they were impressed by the way your complaint system was applied when you invited them to visit your practice and advise about the handling of complaints.

---

This chapter offers some generic cycles of evidence under the headings of consent, confidentiality, and dealing with complaints, to introduce you to the model. Some of them touched on teaching content as well as, or instead of, clinical care but they can be applied to all clinical and non-clinical areas. The following chapters deal in depth with specific areas of teaching and offer examples of evidence cycles on each theme.

# References

1   Chambers R and Wakley G (2000) *Making Clinical Governance Work for You.* Radcliffe Medical Press, Oxford.

2   British Medical Association and Association of British Insurers (2002) *Medical Information and Insurance.* British Medical Association, London (*see* www.bma. org.uk/ap.nsf/Content/MedicalInfoInsurance).

3   General Medical Council (2002) *Seeking Patients' Consent: the ethical considerations.* General Medical Council, London.

4   www.doh.gov.uk/research/.

5   http://www.mencap.org.uk.

6   Royal College of General Practitioners and Brook (2000) *Confidentiality and Young People. A toolkit for general practice, primary care groups and trusts.* Royal College of General Practitioners, London.

7   The Fraser Guidelines (1985) House of Lords Judgement, London.

8   Department of Health (1997) Report of the Review of Patient-identifiable Information. In: *The Caldicott Committee Report.* Department of Health, London.

9   General Medical Council (2003) *Fitness to Practise Statistics for 2002.* General Medical Council, London.

10  Panting G (2003) *Nature of 1000 Claims Against GPs.* Medical Protection Society, London (presentation at primary care conference, Birmingham).

11  MPS Risk Consulting, Granary Wharf House, Leeds LS11 5PY or http://www. mps-riskconsulting.com.

12  MDU Services Ltd, 230 Blackfriars Road, London SE1 8PJ or http://www.the-mdu.com.

# 4

---

# Educational concepts and curriculum development

Healthcare professionals are expected to be 'adult learners'. By this we mean that we will be independent and self-directed to a greater or lesser extent. This can refer both to the way in which we learn and, increasingly with postgraduate study or CPD, the content of what is learnt (the curriculum). This chapter will look at these two areas.

Malcolm Knowles coined the term 'androgogy' to refer to the art and science of teaching adults.[1]

Adult learning theory is built on five assumptions:[1]

- adults are independent and self-directing
- they have accumulated a great deal of experience, which is a rich resource for learning
- they value learning that integrates with the demands of their everyday life
- they are more interested in immediate, problem-centred approaches than in subject-centred ones
- they are more motivated to learn by internal drivers than by external ones.

Medicine, nursing and the allied health professions cover far too big a field for all the content to be delivered by us as teachers. What we need to strive for is to fit our learners with the skills to problem solve and continue learning throughout their careers:

> Education teaches us to solve problems, the nature of which may not be known to us at the time the education is taking place and the solutions to which cannot be seen or even imagined by our teachers.[2]

The capacity to be self-directed however is not an all or nothing function that develops overnight. Learners act at different levels or stages of self-direction depending on many things such as previous teaching, learning and especially assessment experiences, the subject matter and the context of learning. Not all learners are ready to take responsibility for their own learning.

Grow's 'stages of self-directed learning' model proposes four developmental stages for the student (S1–4):[3]

1   dependent learner
2   interested learner
3   involved learner and
4   self-directed learner

and four styles of teaching (T1–4):

1   authority, coach
2   motivator, guide
3   facilitator
4   consultant, delegator.

Effective teachers can match these developmental levels by choosing suitable learning activities. Examples are shown in Table 4.1.

**Table 4.1:**  Stages of self-direction

|         | Student | Teacher | Examples |
|---------|---------|---------|----------|
| Stage 1 | Dependent | Authority, coach | Coaching with immediate feedback<br>Drill<br>Informational lecture<br>Overcoming deficiencies and resistance |
| Stage 2 | Interested | Motivator, guide | Inspiring lecture plus guided discussion<br>Goal setting and learning strategies |
| Stage 3 | Involved | Facilitator | Discussion facilitated by teacher who participates as equal<br>Seminar<br>Group projects |
| Stage 4 | Self-directed | Consultant, delegator | Dissertation<br>Individual work or self-directed study group |

In addition, learners differ in their learning styles – the types of activity that help them to learn best. Effective teachers recognise this and can vary their teaching to suit the learner's preference, whatever the stage of self-directedness of the learner. Learner-centredness is not about leaving the learner to get on with learning entirely on their own but about facilitating that process by knowing how to match what you do as a teacher with learner characteristics.

Knowles further defined seven fundamentals that have stood the test of time as guidelines to encourage adult learners (*see* Box 4.1).[1]

---

**Box 4.1:** Fundamental guidelines to encourage adult learners[1]

1 Establish an effective learning climate where learners feel safe and comfortable expressing themselves.
2 Involve learners in mutual planning of relevant methods and curricular content.
3 Trigger internal motivation by involving learners in diagnosing their own needs.
4 Give learners more control by encouraging them to formulate their own learning objectives.
5 Encourage learners to identify resources and devise strategies for using resources to achieve their objectives.
6 Support learners in carrying out their learning plans.
7 Develop learners' skills of critical reflection by involving learners in evaluating their own learning.

---

Some of the most respected work in relation to adult learners has been done by Brookfield and he also lists six principles of adult learning upon which we can try to build our teaching (*see* Box 4.2).[4]

---

**Box 4.2:** Principles of adult learning[4]

1 Participation is voluntary – the decision to learn is that of the learner.
2 There should be mutual respect – by teachers and learners of each other and by learners of other learners.
3 Collaboration is important – between learners and teachers and among learners.
4 Action and reflection are important – learning is a continuous process of investigation, exploration, action, reflection and further action.
5 Critical reflection brings awareness that alternatives can be presented as challenges to the learner to gather evidence, ask questions and develop a critically aware frame of mind.
6 Self-directed adult individuals need nurturing.

---

Brookfield gave ten tips as to how we might develop our learners to be more adult in their 'approach', which are summarised in Box 4.3.

---

**Box 4.3:**   How to create an adult learner

1   Progressively reduce the learner's dependence on teachers.
2   Help the learner to understand the use of learning resources, including the experiences of others such as fellow learners.
3   Help the learner to use reflective practice to define their learning needs.
4   Help the learner to define their learning objectives, plan their programmes and assess their own progress.
5   Organise what is to be learnt in terms of personal understanding, goals and concerns at the learner's level of understanding.
6   Encourage the learner to take decisions, to expand their learning experiences and range of opportunities for learning.
7   Encourage the use of criteria for judging all aspects of learning and not just those that are easy to measure.
8   Facilitate problem posing and problem solving in relation to personal and group needs issues.
9   Reinforce the concept of the learner as a learner with progressive mastery of skills, through constructive feedback and mutual support.
10  Emphasise experiential learning (learning by doing, learning on the job) and the use of learning contracts.

---

# Curriculum development

The curriculum has been defined as: 'Everything that happens in relation to the educational programme'.[5] The content of what we learn can be formal or informal, planned or unplanned.

Honey and Mumford[6] have commented on the many and varied influences on learning and we can summarise them as shown in Figure 4.1.

Curriculum design, the process of defining and organising learning, should address four areas:

- content
- teaching and learning strategies
- assessment processes
- evaluation processes.

The 'Skilbeck' model[7] of curriculum development includes these important areas and can be drawn as a cycle emphasising the iterative nature of planning and reviewing teaching as in Figure 4.2.

There are four useful questions we can think about when asking what and how we want to learn, both as teachers planning courses or educational opportunities for others, and as learners thinking about our own personal

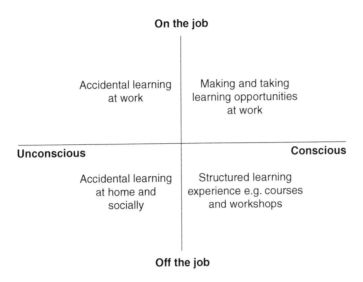

**Figure 4.1:** Sources of learning.

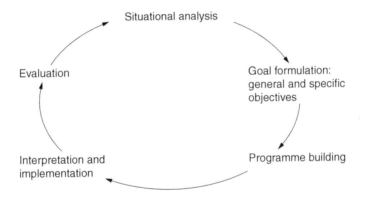

**Figure 4.2:** Curriculum development.

and professional development.[8] These questions take us around Skilbeck's cycle.

- What educational purposes are we seeking to attain?
- What educational experiences are likely to attain those purposes?
- How should we organise those experiences?
- How can we determine whether those purposes are being attained?

# Making a personal learning plan

CPD for individual practitioners introduces a personal element to 'curriculum planning' that very much varies from one person to another and will differ as time goes on. Variations in learning style and personality as well as in experience, interests and job requirements can be taken into account, as people are encouraged to take charge of their learning and development.

Thus, increasingly the principles of self-directedness are being applied to curriculum planning.

# Collecting data to demonstrate your learning, competence, performance and standards of service delivery

## Example cycle of evidence 4.1

- Focus: being learner-centred

---

**Box 4.4:** Case study – being learner-centred is paramount

Jen is running a short day course to update a multidisciplinary group of nurses and doctors and allied health professionals on best practice in the clinical management of back pain. She vows to improve her performance from the last occasion when the participants complained that she and others had lectured at them all day long.

---

This is just an example. Keep your task simple. You could choose three or four cycles of evidence to demonstrate your competence as a teacher each year.

## Stage 1: Select your aspirations for good practice

The excellent healthcare teacher:

- is consistently learner-centred in a variety of teaching situations.

## Stage 2: Set the standards for your outcomes

Outcomes might include:

- a tutorial plan
- mastery of a new skill as a teacher
- a teaching strategy that is implemented
- learner feedback
- evaluation of teaching programmes.

- Feedback, from at least three learners in different situations that confirms that you are learner-centred.

## Stage 3A: Identify your learning needs

- Use a reflective diary: jot down your own perceptions of how learner-centred you are in relation to several learners on different occasions in formal and informal teaching settings.
- Carry out peer review, of the planned curriculum and actual delivery of teaching by an appropriate colleague gauging the extent of learner-centredness and how your approach might be improved.
- Obtain feedback from learners, about the content of your teaching and the match to their own perceived needs, learning styles and preferences.
- Reflect on how you perform compared with the PRISMS model (Product related, Relevant, Interprofessional, Shorter and smaller, Multisite, Symbiotic).[9]

## Stage 3B: Identify your service needs

Any of the needs assessment exercises in 3A may also reveal service needs.

- Use an external review of your teaching, for example, by a training practice assessment, or Quality Assurance Agency including the extent of your learner-centredness in teaching in the workplace.

## Stage 4: Make and carry out a learning and action plan

- Read an original paper about learner-centredness (as in 3A) and discuss with a fellow teacher its implications for improving your teaching practice.
- Write out the curriculum and learning objectives/outcomes for the back pain course for the various participants, according to the requirements of their discipline. Check the course plan against the needs of the participants and the NHS as far as you are able, taking into account the evaluation from the delegates on the last course. Ask an experienced teacher, and others involved in delivery of the course, to review your plan. Revise it accordingly. Reflect on what you have learnt and record it in your own personal development plan.

## Stage 5: Document your learning, competence, performance and standards of service delivery

- Keep a written description, of the changes in the curriculum and delivery of the back pain course to increase learner-centredness. Include the evaluations from the participants.
- Keep a reflective diary, over the time of the task.
- Keep a record of your reflections on original papers on educational strategies and the implications for your own teaching.
- Record feedback and evaluations, from successive groups of learners, including questions on the extent of your learner-centredness.

---

**Box 4.5:**   Case study continued

Jen reacted to the previous dissatisfaction by introducing more interactive sessions including case studies and clinical examinations into the course. She notified the learners in advance so that they knew that they were going to practise clinical examinations on each other.

---

# Example cycle of evidence 4.2

- Focus: teaching and training
- Other relevant focus: clinical care

---

**Box 4.6:** Case study – keeping up to date as a clinical teacher

You have prioritised learning to teach in your personal development plan this year, but you also need to update your clinical knowledge and skills for your everyday work as a health professional. You opt to focus on coronary heart disease (CHD) because of a significant adverse clinical event occurring in your practice or hospital recently.

---

This is just an example. Keep your task simple. You could choose three or four cycles of evidence to demonstrate your competence as a teacher each year.

## Stage 1: Select your aspirations for good practice

The excellent healthcare teacher:

- maintains his or her knowledge and skills, and is aware of his or her limits of competence.

## Stage 2: Set the standards for your outcomes

---

Outcomes might include:

- a tutorial plan
- mastery of a new skill as a teacher
- a teaching strategy that is implemented
- learner feedback
- evaluation of teaching programmes.

---

- An audit of clinical protocol (e.g. CHD) that shows you adhere to best practice.

## Stage 3A: Identify your learning needs

- Use reflective diary observations.
- Compare your own performance against national standards such as the National Service Framework (NSF) standards or those of colleagues or peers elsewhere.
- Undertake a significant event audit – e.g. CHD-related death of 45-year-old male patient.

## Stage 3B: Identify your service needs

Any of the needs assessment exercises in 3A may also reveal service needs.

- Undertake an audit of access to CHD-related diagnostic investigations.
- Compare your current clinical protocol with that recommended by a national body (e.g. the Scottish Intercollegiate Guidelines Network (SIGN) or NICE or other guidelines).

## Stage 4: Make and carry out a learning and action plan

- Learn more about CHD by reviewing evidence (from e.g. Clinical Evidence[10]).
- Find out the expected prevalence in the patient population e.g. from public health department.
- Update a protocol for patient management e.g. for primary/secondary prevention of CHD.
- Attend a masterclass on the clinical topic.

## Stage 5: Document your learning, competence, performance and standards of service delivery

- Keep a reflective diary used in the initial learning needs assessment and after you have completed the learning plan and updated the clinical protocol, to ensure the knowledge gaps have been addressed.
- Keep records of the prevalence of the clinical condition.
- Use the revised clinical protocol and audit to show that your practice is in line with the evidence.
- Keep the minutes of the practice team meeting in which you presented the evidence for the revised practice protocol, and everyone's roles in the updated protocol were agreed.
- Report the significant event audit and how systems were revised as a result.

---

**Box 4.7:** Case study continued

Your learning cycle progresses well. The practice systems for following up patients diagnosed with ischaemic heart disease, and for identifying and assessing those with a family history of heart disease, are tightened up and audited on a regular basis.

---

# Example cycle of evidence 4.3

- Focus: teaching and training

---

**Box 4.8:** Case study – adapting to differing learning styles

Ann is apprehensive about teaching the group of junior doctors at their induction. They are expected to learn about what the trust expects concerning human resource matters including their working hours and other employee issues. She realises that to engage the attention of the doctors, she needs to provide the information in a variety of ways to appeal to the doctors' differing learning styles.

---

This is just an example. Keep your task simple. You could choose three or four cycles of evidence to demonstrate your competence as a teacher each year.

## *Stage 1: Select your aspirations for good practice*

The excellent healthcare teacher:

- uses teaching methods appropriate to the learning styles of those participating in the educational activity.

## *Stage 2: Set the standards for your outcomes*

---

Outcomes might include:

- a tutorial plan
- mastery of a new skill as a teacher
- a teaching strategy that is implemented
- learner feedback
- evaluation of teaching programmes.

---

- Learners gain and apply new knowledge and skills under your guidance.
- Develop an understanding of others' learning styles; develop a flexible strategy for teaching others with different learning styles.

## Stage 3A: Identify your learning needs

- Keep a reflective diary, recording your account of teaching learners during teaching sessions and answering their queries on an everyday basis.
- Use peer review of an audiotape or videotape of yourself conducting a tutorial.

## Stage 3B: Identify your service needs

> Any of the needs assessment exercises in 3A may also reveal service needs.

- Review whether the learning needs of all those for whom you are responsible for teaching have been identified over the last 6–12 months, and are known to you, before you embark on teaching them in a formal or informal capacity.
- Undertake a SWOT analysis with the line managers or educational supervisors of learners to determine whether sufficient resources are provided for the teaching methods appropriate to learning styles and the educational objectives.

## Stage 4: Make and carry out a learning and action plan

- Read up on Honey and Mumford's learning styles.[6]
- Observe an 'expert' teacher at work with a diverse group of students. Discuss the way he/she adapted to differing learning styles and the response from the students.
- Review the audio or videotape with a peer (see Stage 3A above).
- Present your results from the SWOT analysis to the trust and/or deanery to discuss how resources for teaching can be extended.

## Stage 5: Document your learning, competence, performance and standards of service delivery

- Repeat your observations in your reflective diary in relation to all teaching and training activities.
- Repeat the SWOT analysis after changes have been made.

- Compare audits of a learner's practice before and after the learner has participated in a teaching session with you.
- Retain the lesson plan and notes from a teaching session recording the adaptations made to accommodate differing styles of learning, together with the feedback from the students.

---

**Box 4.9:** Case study continued

After learning more about other people's learning styles, Ann arranges her session to include a large group discussion about the human resources topics, small group problem solving around examples of common issues for doctors, and a handout with facts and figures.

---

# References

1 Knowles MS (1984) *Androgogy in Action: applying modern principles of adult learning.* Jossey-Bass, San Francisco.

2 Marinker M (1992) Assessment of postgraduate medical education – future directions. In: M Lawrence and P Pritchard (eds) *General Practice Education UK and Nordic Perspectives.* Springer Verlag London, Goldaming, Surrey.

3 Grow GO (1996) Teaching learners to be self-directed. *Adult Education Quarterly.* **41 (3)**: 125–49.

4 Brookfield SD (1986) *Understanding and Facilitating Adult Learning.* Open University Press, Milton Keynes.

5 Glenn JM (1995) *Course Materials.* Dundee University, Centre for Medical Education, Dundee.

6 www.peterhoney.com.

7 Skilbeck M (1975) School based curriculum development and teacher education. (Mimeograph) cited by H Mulholland (1988) in *Curriculum Design and Development.* Centre for Medical Education, University of Dundee, Dundee.

8 Prideaux D (2003) Curriculum design. In: ABC of learning and teaching in medicine. *British Medical Journal.* **326**: 268–70.

9 Bligh J (2001) Product related, Relevant, Interprofessional, Shorter and smaller, Multisite, Symbiotic (PRISMS): new educational strategies for medical education. *Medical Education.* **35**: 520–1.

10 www.clinicalevidence.com.

# Further reading

- Gerald Grow (Professor of Journalism at Florida A and M University, Tallahassee, USA). More about the stages of self-directed learning model and other works can be found at: www.longleaf.net/ggrow.

# 5

## Matching methods of teaching with your message

This chapter considers several teaching strategies with tips for making the best use of them.

In considering which teaching method to use, try asking yourself the following questions:

- what am I trying to achieve, what are my objectives?
- what are the learners' objectives?
- is this the best way of achieving them?
- what other ways are there of achieving them?
- what are the strengths of the way I have chosen?
- what are the potential weaknesses that I will have to be on guard for as a facilitator?
- how will I know that this way is the most appropriate way – for me and my learners?
- how will I assess whether the objectives have been achieved?

## Tips for *ad hoc* teaching

Much healthcare teaching is done in the clinic or by the bedside with little time to prepare. You can still however prepare a structure in advance that helps you to be more effective. The one given in Box 5.1 is adapted from *The One Minute Preceptor: five microskills for clinical teaching.*[1]

**Box 5.1:** Five microskills for clinical teaching

1   *Get a commitment.* Ask, 'what do you think is going on here?' Asking the trainee how they interpreted the situation is the first step in diagnosing their learning needs.
2   *Probe for supporting evidence.* Ask, 'what led you to that conclusion?' Ask the trainee for their evidence before offering your opinion. This will allow you to find out about what they know and identify where they have gaps.
3   *Teach general rules and principles.* 'When this happens, do this ...' Instruction will be remembered better if in the form of a general rule or principle.
4   *Reinforce what was right and be specific.* 'You did an excellent job of ...' Skills in learners that are not well established need to be reinforced, and remember that praise motivates.
5   *Correct mistakes.* 'Next time this happens try this instead ...' Mistakes that are left unattended have a good chance of being repeated.

# Tips for teaching a practical skill

The three basic elements of a practical teaching session are:

1   preparation (set)
2   procedure (dialogue)
3   summary (closure).

## Preparation (set)

- Define precise objectives.
- Identify the association of the skill with other learning events.
- Decide what form the teaching will take.
- Plan the environment e.g. location, lighting, seating, positioning and equipment – check function.

Ensure that the learner is familiar with the arrangements and knows what you are going to do before the teaching session begins.

## Procedure (dialogue)[2]

There are two components to this, the learning of the skill and the discussion. The discussion will usually include an element of feedback.

- The teacher performs the procedure without commentary, at normal speed.
- The teacher talks the procedure through; the teacher performs the procedure.

- The learner talks the procedure through; the teacher performs the procedure.
- The learner talks the procedure through; the learner performs the procedure.

## Summary (closure)

- Reflection/critique/feedback using Pendleton's principles.[3]
- Questions.
- Plan next session.

# Tips for giving effective lectures

- Research your audience.
- Practise and time your talk – get feedback from colleagues if possible.
- Think about how your talk fits with what else the learners are considering.
- Open your lecture by sparking the attention of the audience in some way – with a prop, a challenging remark or a rhetorical question. Do not open by apologising for your lack of knowledge or for being there or keeping them from food, drink, or freedom.
- 'Say what you are going to say, say it and then repeat what you said', as they say.
- Arrive early – check equipment.
- Take your own pointer.
- Fix your notes together and/or number the pages.
- Use a highlighter pen for your lecture notes.
- Include the whole audience by scanning them with your eyes.
- Develop your own style. Don't try and be funny if telling jokes makes you quake or you are hopeless at delivering the punchline. Don't be crude or swear in a professional setting.
- Wear comfortable clothes.
- Have some water standing by.
- Write yourself big notices saying 'slow down' if you tend to speak too fast; put timings in big letters in your lecture notes if you tend to slow down.
- Keep an eye on the time throughout.
- Let the audience know if they can interrupt you with questions.
- Think positive and exude an air of enthusiasm and confidence about the subject.
- Finish with a well-polished relevant conclusion; it might be the answer to the rhetorical question posed at the beginning, the end of a story half told earlier in the presentation, a challenge or an action plan for the future.

# Tips for running a workshop

- Choose an unambiguous title.
- Circulate abstracts and the backgrounds of the facilitators.
- Hold a practice session.
- Plan a timetable.
- Know who is in the group and how many.
- Have enough handouts.
- Check flip chart paper, pens and blue tack.
- Keep any small group presenters reporting back focused on presenting the discussion of their tasks.
- Round up the final plenary discussion with a conclusion based on the small group discussions that relates back to the objectives of the workshop.

# Tips for small group working

- Limit the numbers to fewer than 12.
- Place chairs in a circle to help all members to feel equally part of the group.
- Remove any empty chairs so that the group feels complete.
- Appoint a facilitator who is skilled at handling group dynamics.
- Welcome everybody and check introductions.
- Insist on respect and confidentiality within the group.
- Clarify the task.
- Ensure facilitators keep the group to task.
- Appoint a reporter other than the facilitator to report the group's discussion to the plenary.
- Facilitate, don't act as instructor.
- Ensure that everyone contributes.
- Keep to time.

Consider using 'talking walls', an 'active photograph', the 'goldfish bowl technique' or 'trios' to enliven a small group and encourage active participation or extend the small group to a learning group over time.[4]

# Tips for using problem-based learning

Problem-based learning (PBL) reverses the traditional approach to teaching and learning. It starts with individual examples or problems; by considering these learners develop general principles and concepts that they can generalise to other situations.[5]

It can foster deep learning, requires students to activate prior learning and integrate new learning with it and can develop lifelong learning skills and generic competencies such as collaboration.

---

**Box 5.2:**   How to create effective PBL scenarios

- Define learning objectives in advance.
- Problems should be appropriate to the stage of the curriculum and the level of learner understanding.
- Scenarios should be relevant to practice.
- Problems should be presented in context to encourage integration of knowledge.
- Scenarios should present cues to stimulate discussion and encourage learners to seek an explanation.
- The problem should be of sufficient depth to prevent too early resolution.
- Students should be actively engaged in searching for information.

---

Consider the example in Table 5.1:

**Table 5.1:**   Example of steps in the problem-based learning process

| The problem | Group discussion |
| --- | --- |
| The mother of a 13-year-old girl phones the surgery to ask the receptionist whether her daughter has been seen that day by a doctor. | The group clarifies the text of the problem scenario. |
| Isn't that confidential information? | Learners define the problem. |
| She is underage, the mother must be worried. The girl might never come again if she thinks we tell her mother everything. Should that be something the receptionist deals with or the doctor? | Brainstorming is used to identify possible explanations/solutions. |
| It's an ethical/medico-legal dilemma. | The group reaches an interim conclusion. |
| To find out what the law says. To find out what ethicists think. To find out what doctors say in real life. | The group formulates learning objectives. |
| Library visits, internet searches, interviews with practitioners, discussion among peers, friends and family are needed. | The learners go away and work independently to achieve the learning outcomes. |
| Pooling of results and sources is required. The tutor checks learning, clarifies and corrects if necessary. | The group reconvenes to discuss the knowledge acquired. |

## Disadvantages of PBL[6]

- Students can feel 'all at sea' if the process is not managed and introduced well. Learners learn as they are taught (and assessed) and most are not prepared for such a high degree of self-directedness.
- Tutors may not have the competencies to manage PBL – taught as they were in a traditional curriculum.
- Tutors may resent not being able to 'teach' i.e. transfer their knowledge and understanding.
- Knowledge gained can tend to be disorganised and the important points not distinguished from the unimportant. Good tutoring is required to address this at the last stage.
- More staff and resources may be needed to support and facilitate the session and the searches.
- Students may miss out on role modelling from inspirational teachers.

Many of these can be addressed through training and preparation, of learners and tutors.


# Tips for using computer-supported learning

## Advantages of computer-based learning

- Access to a huge amount of information is possible, linking resources in different formats.
- It allows and supports flexible delivery, distance learning, workplace-based learning.
- Learners can follow the course materials at their own pace, independently, actively and in a way that suits their learning needs.
- Interactivity, attractive animations and simulations can be built into design course materials as easily as less stimulating, traditional materials.
- Discussion forums (email, video-conferencing, live lectures, virtual learning environments) can be set up for learner support, collaboration and development.
- Self-assessments can be built in for students to monitor their own progress – giving quick feedback and freeing up tutors from excessive individual involvement.

## Disadvantages of computer-based learning

- Learners need access to the technology and appropriate skills to use it.
- The role of the inspirational teacher as role model and motivator might be lost in fully web-based courses.
- Learners like to meet other 'real' people for face-to-face contact.
- Web-based learning favours self-starters and those able to work alone.
- Learners may need to be guided to important, reliable information and require high powers of discrimination or critical appraisal of the literature.
- It may require specialist technical support to prepare and use.
- Slow systems cause frustration as downloading of videos and images hold up learning.
- It can be difficult to authenticate individual students' work.

# Collecting data to demonstrate your learning, competence, performance and standards of service delivery

## Example cycle of evidence 5.1

- Focus: teaching and training
- Other relevant focus: relationships with patients

---

**Box 5.3:** Case study – teaching patients by appropriate means

Lesley and Francis are planning to run a roadshow for patients about preventing heart disease. As health promotion facilitators, they have devised a one-hour session that can be run from any health setting in their locality. They need to be able to engage their audience and hold their attention, and be flexible in relation to the needs of people attending, with the right audiovisual aids.

---

This is just an example. Keep your task simple. You could choose three or four cycles of evidence to demonstrate your competence as a teacher each year.

*Stage 1: Select your aspirations for good practice*

The excellent healthcare teacher:

- uses clear language appropriate for patients
- gives patients the information they need about their problem in a way they can understand
- takes time to listen to patients and allow them to express their concerns.

*Stage 2: Set the standards for your outcomes*

Outcomes might include:

- a tutorial plan
- mastery of a new skill as a teacher
- a teaching strategy that is implemented
- learner feedback
- evaluation of teaching programmes.

- Construct information aids for patients reflecting best practice in a clinical topic.
- Good consultation and communication skills with patients that enable you to motivate them to adopt healthy lifestyles.

*Stage 3A: Identify your learning needs*

- Undertake a patient feedback quiz to find out if patients who have attended the roadshow are well informed about their clinical conditions.
- Ask nurse colleagues for their views on whether the patient's understanding of the clinical condition had improved after attending the roadshow. Ask specifically for feedback about the clarity of information you gave to patients and extent to which you have explained risks in clear and understandable ways.

*Stage 3B: Identify your service needs*

Any of the needs assessment exercises in 3A may also reveal service needs.

- Use a quiz at the roadshow to determine the extent to which patients have unanswered questions despite having consulted local healthcare colleagues.

- Ask for feedback from a patient participation group or forum about what resources they want, but perceive as being unavailable, for helping patients to stop smoking, lose weight etc.

## Stage 4: Make and carry out a learning and action plan

- Learn about appropriate and effective ways of giving information to patients by reviewing relevant literature.
- Obtain literature from patients' organisations about effective ways to provide information.
- Meet with nurse colleagues to discuss information needs of patients with CHD, those with a family history of CHD and those whose risk for CHD is unknown.

## Stage 5: Document your learning, competence, performance and standards of service delivery

- Keep results from a questionnaire completed by patients to show that their information needs have been met.
- Conduct a re-audit of patients' attempts to comply with advice you gave.
- Make notes on the teaching points about best practice in the giving of patient information, together with examples of appropriate patient information leaflets.
- Copy of an information leaflet and decision-making aids for patients that have been adopted by a general practice.

---

**Box 5.4:**   Case study continued

Lesley and Francis received fantastic feedback from patients as they varied the way they delivered their health messages depending on the nature of those attending their roadshows. They used video and interactive CD ROMs, and had interactive software that allowed those attending to visualise their risk of consequences of CHD and how this might be lessened by reducing their risk factors.

---

# Example cycle of evidence 5.2

- Focus: teaching and training

---

**Box 5.5:**   Case study – teaching a practical skill

Prasad is a GP with a special interest (GPwSI) in musculoskeletal orthopaedics. Part of his job is to teach joint injection techniques to other GPs, nurses with a special interest in rheumatology and senior house officers who are new to rheumatology. He often has a practitioner with him during his clinics and has to be ready to take any opportunity to teach these learners about joint injections or other aspects of rheumatology in the busy clinic.

---

This is just an example. Keep your task simple. You could choose three or four cycles of evidence to demonstrate your competence each year.

## Stage 1: Select your aspirations for good practice

The excellent healthcare teacher:

- is able to optimise the learning experience of the student while teaching a practical skill, by facilitating the learner in preparing for observing and/or practising the procedure
- minimises or avoids risk to the patient while the student learns a new practical skill.

## Stage 2: Set the standards for your outcomes

---

Outcomes might include:

- a tutorial plan
- mastery of a new skill as a teacher
- a teaching strategy that is implemented
- learner feedback
- evaluation of teaching programmes.

---

- Define the teaching objectives.
- Check that the student can perform the practical skill in line with best practice without supervision.
- Ensure the service is organised to maximise learning opportunities.

## Stage 3A: Identify your learning needs

- Arrange a peer review by a colleague with expertise in the practical skill that you are teaching. Look for the extent to which you explain the procedure, perform it in line with best practice, and facilitate others in discussion of the procedure and its practice.
- Obtain feedback from those to whom you are teaching the practical skill. Ask what went well, what might be improved, their level of confidence when undertaking the procedure for the first time, when supervised and unsupervised, and if they felt able to ask questions.
- Undertake a risk assessment of the teaching of the procedure to learner groups, including an assessment of the range of their prior experience, qualifications, knowledge and skills.

## Stage 3B: Identify your service needs

> Any of the needs assessment exercises in 3A may also reveal service needs.

- Obtain patient feedback from those who have had the procedure while you were teaching. Include the giving of informed consent, the communication or consultation skills of practitioners, pain control, the opportunities to ask questions, the information given, etc.[7]
- Audit the success of the procedure undertaken by each operator. Measure the result depending on nature of the procedure (e.g. the infection rate, relief of pain, histology reports, etc.).
- Ask for a report by the newly skilled practitioners of their capacity to practise the new skills. Include the availability of support staff or equipment, referrals from other practitioners, funding from organisation for service, etc.

## Stage 4: Make and carry out a learning and action plan

- Make a video of yourself teaching the procedure to learners (with informed consent from patients and learners). Comment on your own performance or discuss with a colleague who has expertise in teaching and/or the practice of the procedure.

- Find out more about best practice in executing the procedure or improving the environment for teaching. You might look for potential technology or modern equipment, lighting, positioning of equipment, alternative techniques. You could search for new information from the Royal Colleges' websites, from the literature by obtaining and reading published papers, or by visiting other departments where the procedure is performed to compare approaches.
- Find out about best practice in informed consent in relation to teaching and in respect of making the video recording. Obtain a template for the video consent form from, for example, the RCGP.[8]

### *Stage 5: Document your learning, competence, performance and standards of service delivery*

- Make a video of a teaching session (retained for a limited period as specified on patient consent form) and document the critique or reflections.
- Keep a signed video consent form.
- Collect feedback from peers, patients and/or learners.
- Audit the results from following up a newly skilled practitioner's performance of procedure.
- Conduct a risk assessment of learners undertaking the procedure.

---

**Box 5.6:**   Case study continued

Prasad put a great deal of effort into preparing the learners for undertaking the practical procedure of joint injection, by allowing them to observe him performing the procedure, then talking them through it, then the learner talking him through it while Prasad undertook the injection, before they performed their first procedure. With this approach learners did not have any problem becoming competent in joint injections.

---

# Example cycle of evidence 5.3

- Focus: problem-based learning

---

**Box 5.7:**   Case study – problem-based learning

Carl has been appointed as the PBL tutor at the local university where a medical school has just been established. His job is to teach and support local GPs and primary care nurses in using the PBL approach for the medical students who will be placed in the community for a good proportion of their time. Carl is aware that the way he teaches and supports colleague teachers in PBL facilitation skills is critical to their enablement of medical students' learning, and the reputation of the medical school.

---

> This is just an example. Keep your task simple. You could choose three or four cycles of evidence to demonstrate your competence as a teacher each year.

## Stage 1: Select your aspirations for good practice

The excellent healthcare teacher who uses PBL:

- understands the PBL process
- has skills to encourage the self-directed learning crucial for the students' progress.

## Stage 2: Set the standards for your outcomes

---

Outcomes might include:

- a tutorial plan
- mastery of a new skill as a teacher
- a teaching strategy that is implemented
- learner feedback
- evaluation of teaching programmes.

---

- PBL is used appropriately to meet the learning objectives.
- The use of PBL optimises the extent and depth of the students' learning.

## Stage 3A: Identify your learning needs

- Check out if you are sufficiently familiar with the process of PBL. You could write down the steps of the process and compare yours with the suggested stages on page 79.
- Write out three scenarios that you believe are suitable for PBL and ask your PBL tutor to critique your efforts and suggest revisions. Ask the tutor to comment on whether the learning objectives and problems are relevant, the problems are appropriate to curriculum and stage of learner, and whether there is sufficient context and depth.
- Ask any students who you have supervised doing PBL to give you feedback in informal or formal ways about the process, the scenario, your facilitation, and the overall outcomes.

## Stage 3B: Identify your service needs

> Any of the needs assessment exercises in 3A may also reveal service needs.

- Compare the feedback from students about various teachers' facilitation skills and understanding of the process.
- Measure facets of students' learning and students' engagement; compare them against the learning objectives, the organisation of learning, the availability of information sources and the evidence to solve the problems. Look for reasons why students' experiences and learning outcomes might differ – in relation to a particular teacher, the circumstances of the student or the time spent.

## Stage 4: Make and carry out a learning and action plan

- Carrying out exercises in sections 3A and 3B will be an integral part of learning.
- Read up about PBL and competencies of problem-based tutors.[5,6,9]
- Attend a workshop on the teaching of PBL and any support group for PBL tutors.

*Stage 5: Document your learning, competence, performance and standards of service delivery*

- Collect workshop notes, certificates of attendance and outstanding training needs in your continuing PDP.
- Record the needs assessment and learning from the first two exercises of 3A with corrections and revisions to the list of steps in the PBL process and PBL scenarios.
- Obtain feedback from students engaged in PBL under your tutorship.
- Give a checklist of your current or achieved competencies versus those recommended by researchers giving the reference of the research study.

---

**Box 5.8:**   Case study continued

The students are enthusiastic about the PBL approach thanks to the excellent facilitation skills of GPs and primary care nurses who are well versed in the PBL process. The medical students rate the scenarios highly. The electronic and paper-based documents and books accessed at the university and postgraduate centre libraries prove to be great resources for finding information about best evidence.

---

# References

1  Gordon K, Meyer B and Irby D (1992) *The One Minute Preceptor: five microskills for clinical teaching.* University of Washington, Seattle, USA.

2  Peyton JWR (1998) *Teaching and Learning in Medical Practice.* Manticore Europe Ltd, Rickmansworth.

3  Pendleton D, Schofield T, Tate P and Havelock P (1984) *The Consultation, an Approach to Teaching and Learning.* Oxford Medical Publications, Oxford.

4  Mohanna K, Chambers R and Wall D (2003) *Teaching Made Easy* (2e). Radcliffe Medical Press, Oxford.

5  Davis MH and Harden RM (1999) *Problem Based Learning: a practical guide.* AMEE Education guide 15. Centre for Medical Education, Dundee.

6  Wood D (2003) Problem based learning. ABC of learning and teaching in medicine. *British Medical Journal.* **326**: 328–30.

7  Tate P (2001) *The Doctors' Communication Handbook.* Radcliffe Medical Press, Oxford.

8  Chambers R (2002) *A Guide to Accredited Professional Development.* Royal College of General Practitioners, London.

9  Naidoo S and Dennick R (2003) The implementation and evaluation of problem-based learning on a vocational training scheme for general practice registrars. *Education for Primary Care.* **14**: 178–88.

# 6

# Organising educational activities

Good organisation and preparation is key to getting the most out of any educational activity for more than one reason. Meeting organisers should feel that they have a serious duty of care for potential delegates to ensure that time will not be wasted by attending the course or conference. That not only means providing quality education but also double checking every stage in the organisation of the event to make sure that everything runs smoothly and that nothing is left to chance.

In addition, the first of the foundations for adult learning as identified by Knowles is to establish the physical and psychological climate or ethos for learning.[1] That requires teachers to pay attention to all aspects of the 'educational environment'. Consider the following:

> The crucial knowledge concerns the overall atmosphere or characteristics of the classroom; the kind of things that are rewarded, encouraged, emphasised; the style of life that is valued in the classroom or school community and is most visibly expressed and felt.[2]

The educational environment is important in the healthcare professions in the way that it can encourage less well-defined behaviours such as 'professionalism' or 'bedside manner'. By ensuring attention to aspects of the learning environment and offering ourselves as role models, teachers can contribute to the likelihood that such behaviours will be fostered.

Ask yourself the questions in Box 6.1 in relation to the educational environment you cultivate for your learners.

---

**Box 6.1:** CUES to the educational environment (College and University Environment Scales)[2]

- *Scholarship*: as a teacher, what am I doing to encourage scholarly, intellectual and academic pursuits?
- *Practicality*: how much attention do I give to the pragmatic and the practical, business-like efficiency?
- *Community*: is there concern about the fostering of friendliness and a sense of community between teacher and students and among students?
- *Awareness*: what do I do that might encourage the development of a sense of personal identity and self-expression and foster a sense of social responsibility?
- *Propriety*: to what extent do I place emphasis on the environment being a polite and considerate sort of place, where 'proper' behaviours are called for and where there is some emphasis on taking note of rules and regulations?

---

# Writing educational materials

A key aspect of the organisation of any learning activity is the provision of written materials. Any learning activity will be enhanced if attention is given to providing written information that is easy to use and well presented.

Course materials, handouts for those attending presentations or courses, or patient information leaflets are all part of teaching and there are a few simple rules for effective writing:

- write in clear, simple language
- use short sentences
- don't use two-syllable words if there is a one-syllable option
- pitch the content at the right level for the reader
- make the layout attractive with plenty of white space
- include boxes for key points
- use subheadings to break up the text
- add illustrations and diagrams to complement the text
- focus on relevant material rather than rambling anecdotes
- explain any jargon or abbreviations.

---

**Box 6.2:** Make a plan for your writing

- Introduction to include definitions, objectives.
- Main themes: usually three, four or five.
- Discussion.
- Conclusions.
- Further ideas.
- References.
- Sources of further information.

---

# Use of handouts

The amount and type of information in a handout will depend on why you are providing written information in addition to requiring attendance at the teaching session.

On the whole there are three main teacher-centred reasons for handouts:

1   to provide a place for learners to take notes alongside an outline of the session, ensuring that they have all the important information
2   to provide extra detail or information that would detract from the flow of the lecture, but that learners need to be able to make sense of what is being presented, such as reports, figures or tables
3   to provide extra information such as vignettes for case discussion or for small group work.

And there are three main learner-centred reasons:

1   as an aide-mémoire, maybe for revision for exams, of what was said with personal annotations of what was interesting or seemed important
2   as a record of what was said to prevent having to take notes and thus to aid concentration
3   as a record of what was said to prevent having to take notes – or even attend.

A handout should capture the key points of your talk or workshop but need not be too comprehensive as those who are particularly interested in the topic can follow up your session with private reading. A further reading list or references to key literature or sources of further information is a very useful inclusion in a handout.

The rules of copyright preclude you from photocopying large sections of published work for dissemination to students unless the publishers have printed their express permission that their book's contents are fully photocopyable. This has implications if you are teaching critical reading skills and wish to provide copies of journals for the session. Handouts in advance of such a session might usefully give the reference so that students can bring it along themselves – and they may even read it in preparation! You are usually allowed to copy about 5% of a literary work for your own research or private study. You may be able to obtain the publisher's permission to provide photocopies of specific articles for students if you write and ask, or pay a copying fee by arrangement.

The reasons for providing handouts will govern not only what they contain but also the time at which you give them out.

•   Handouts given beforehand allow preparation or homework, can set the scene or allow problems to be identified.

- Handouts given at the start of a session can distract the audience who may spend time reading them and not listening.
- Handouts not given until the end cannot be annotated and personalised, but ...
- If not given until the end students are 'persuaded' against leaving early.
- If handouts are given out at the start, time should be given for learners to look at and be aware of the content so that they will recognise new information in the lecture that might need to be noted down.
- Some learners need to know if handouts are to be issued so that they can listen at a different level – maybe reflective learners will not concentrate on detail that they can read later, but on making internal maps and integrating this new information with that which they already have.
- Handouts with activities or interactivity, such as completing the blanks, can promote active learning.

Table 6.1 lists examples of common things that can go wrong when organising educational events and gives a few suggestions to minimise that possibility.

**Table 6.1:**   Common things that can go wrong when organising educational events and how to minimise problems

| *Things that can go wrong when organising educational events:* | *Safeguard against them happening by:* |
| --- | --- |
| Too few people apply and you have to cancel the conference, course or seminar. | • Market research<br>• Good advertising |
| Speakers fail to turn up at a conference or course. | • Organising travel or accommodation<br>• Sending reminders and maps<br>• Giving plenty of notice<br>• Making sure pay is appropriate |
| Delegates arrive late at a course as travelling there took them longer than expected or they lost their way. | • Choosing the venue carefully<br>• Sending maps<br>• Ensuring good signposting |
| You keep delegates working flat out and deprive them of the opportunity to take advantage of their surroundings, despite having chosen the isolated location for the course because of its sporting facilities or rural situation. | • Ensure a balanced, not too packed, programme<br>• Recognising that learners need time to reflect and take in what they are learning as well as to network with other learners |
| You circulate paperwork to delegates after the course because you or the speakers had not prepared or been able to give out the appropriate handouts at the event. | • Requesting handouts from speakers in advance<br>• Considering posting them on the web |

*continued opposite*

**Table 6.1:**   *continued*

| *Things that can go wrong when organising educational events:* | *Safeguard against them happening by:* |
| --- | --- |
| Speakers are booked for their convenient availability rather than because they are the most appropriate lecturers for the required level of knowledge or topic. | • Planning well in advance and inviting speakers early – up to a year ahead |
| You run a course or conference to fulfil your own educational needs or preferences rather than those of the intended audience. | • Conducting needs assessment exercises<br>• Involving learners in planning |
| You choose a lecture format as an easier option than other methods of delivery, resulting in a disappointing educational event for the delegates with few opportunities for asking questions and developing ideas on a topic that needed interactive discussion and reflection. | • Setting clear objectives<br>• Matching the most appropriate method to achieve these objectives |
| The administration of a correspondence course is disorganised so that successive modules are sent out late with significant delays in answering queries or marking completed work. | • Learning to let go – employ someone efficient and with the time to do the administration effectively |
| Teachers become swamped with teaching, giving feedback or support or marking assessments | • Asking whether the course is too teacher-centred? Consider a more 'teacher-light' strategy and devolve responsibility for learning to the learners |

---

**Box 6.3:**

For any educational activity, learning will be enhanced by:

- *adequate preparation and checking* – of budget, sponsorship, venue, transport/parking, speakers, visual aids, catering, facilities
- *explicit objective setting* – what is the purpose of the session, who is it relevant to, do they need pre-course preparation/reading?
- *activity selection* – what sort of session would achieve these objectives most effectively?
- *thorough evaluation* – what went well, why, what changes are needed for next time?

# Collecting data to demonstrate your learning, competence, performance and standards of service delivery

## Example cycle of evidence 6.1

- Focus: teaching and learning
- Other relevant focus: working with colleagues

---

**Box 6.4:**   Case study – keeping learning as interactive as possible

Keiran is organising the annual updating workshop for vocational trainers in dentistry. The dentists who attended last year have asked him to make sure that it is as interactive as possible. The previous workshop had involved six hour-long lectures and little else. Having discussed the objectives of the day with his boss at the deanery, he concludes that they need to start with a formal presentation from the dental dean to let everyone know about any changes in regulations and new systems in the deanery. After that, the rest of the day should revolve around small group work, as the purpose of the day is for the participants to discuss good practice and experiences, generate new ideas for the deanery and challenge current thinking, reflect on their own training role, and share their feelings or problems.

---

This is just an example. Keep your task simple. You could choose three or four cycles of evidence to demonstrate your competence as a teacher each year.

*Stage 1: Select your aspirations for good practice*

The excellent healthcare teacher:

- is able to match the method of delivering their teaching with the purpose of the learning, taking account of learners' needs and circumstances.

## *Stage 2: Set the standards for your outcomes*

Outcomes might include:

- a tutorial plan
- mastery of a new skill as a teacher
- a teaching strategy that is implemented
- learner feedback
- evaluation of teaching programmes.

- Be able to deliver teaching by a variety of methods in order to optimise opportunities for others to learn and produce intended outcomes from the teaching session.

## *Stage 3A: Identify your learning needs*

- Draw up a list of methods of teaching with which you are familiar and circumstances in which they might be the preferred method or might be disadvantageous. Read more about methods in other books and add them to the list.[3] Look for new methods with which you were previously unfamiliar or new perspectives on how to use known methods.
- Undertake a SWOT analysis of all methods of teaching you and a 'buddy' (*see* page 23) or teaching colleague use. Ask an experienced tutor to comment on the conclusions of your SWOT analysis in the light of his/her own experience.
- Use peer review or structured feedback from the participants attending your teaching sessions, especially if, as in the case study, those attending your teaching sessions are teachers themselves and can give you well-informed feedback. You might even run a teaching session in the updating day of the case study to critique methods used in that day workshop.

## *Stage 3B: Identify your service needs*

Any of the needs assessment exercises in 3A may also reveal service needs.

- Run a nominal group exercise so that everyone contributes their thoughts about the way the usual delivery of teaching in their organisation could be improved.

- Prepare scenarios to be used in trios. In the scenarios, the task of the teacher is to give information about a specific subject and to determine the extent of the learner's knowledge from the feedback; the observer records how well this is done. Then have a large group feedback to draw conclusions about what techniques worked.

### Stage 4: Make and carry out a learning and action plan

- Undertaking the exercises in sections 3A and 3B will constitute much of your learning plan.
- Attend an accredited postgraduate teaching programme to learn more about effective teaching and develop expertise in a wider variety of teaching methods. You can then be more flexible in matching your method of teaching with the messages you have planned to convey.

### Stage 5: Document your learning, competence, performance and standards of service delivery

- Prepare notes capturing the content and your reflections of SWOT analysis.
- List the methods of delivery of teaching together with the advantages and disadvantages and the circumstances in which they are the preferred method.
- Record the conclusions from nominal group exercise and subsequent action plan for improvements.
- Record the conclusions from the trio work in the second part of 3B.

---

**Box 6.5:**    Case study continued

The updating day went really well and there was a real buzz from the networking and exchange of ideas and sharing of solutions for each other's problems. The feedback showed that dentists participating were appreciative of the way that Keiran had organised the programme and nearly everyone thought that there had been sufficient time for discussion. Several participants suggested holding a similar event in six months' time rather than waiting for another year to go by as they had got so much out of the day.

---

# Example cycle of evidence 6.2

- Focus: creating a learning organisation

---

**Box 6.6:**   Case study – creating and sustaining a learning organisation

Theresa has had a sideways move into another trust. One of the first things she notices is the real commitment of her new trust to becoming a 'learning organisation'. They are actively trying to turn the rhetoric into reality and create a working environment throughout the trust that encourages learning, for the entire workforce. Line managers are role models for their staff. All staff, including doctors, nurses, allied health professionals, managers and support staff, have PDPs that are reviewed annually as well as appraisals. The budget for education and training is sufficient for the majority of course fees and cover that have been prioritised from personal reviews or anticipated from service changes and there is regular protected time for learning as organisation-wide or workplace events.

---

This is just an example. Keep your task simple. You could choose three or four cycles of evidence to demonstrate your competence as a teacher each year.

## Stage 1: Select your aspirations for good practice
The excellent healthcare teacher:

- cultivates an educational environment for learners.

## Stage 2: Set the standards for your outcomes

---

Outcomes might include:

- a tutorial plan
- mastery of a new skill as a teacher
- a teaching strategy that is implemented
- learner feedback
- evaluation of teaching programmes.

---

- Create a working environment throughout the organisation that encourages learning.
- Create sufficient opportunities for all members of the workforce for their personal and organisational needs and priorities.

### Stage 3A: Identify your learning needs

- Self-assess whether you know the essential components of a learning organisation.[4]
- Invite suggestions from those you teach or for whom you organise a programme of educational events about what you might reorganise or establish so your teaching is more conducive to their learning.
- Discuss your own PDP at a regular review with a CPD tutor or at appraisal. Listen to the views of your colleagues and the suggestions about your own progress in your PDP and how you have addressed your learning needs and made changes in practice. Consider if there are barriers to your own learning and change in your workplace or organisation that also apply to others working there and if there are ways to overcome those barriers for the good of everyone.

### Stage 3B: Identify your service needs

Any of the needs assessment exercises in 3A may also reveal service needs.

- Discuss with staff who have changed their roles and responsibilities whether they think that they have sufficient knowledge and skills to be competent in their post. Establish if they needed and received training to render them competent before taking on the new roles.
- Compare the approach to learning in your workplace or the wider organisation with best practice in establishing and sustaining a learning organisation – use checklist of best practice to give an overarching view.[4]

### Stage 4: Make and carry out a learning and action plan

- Read up about the meaning of the term learning organisation, and the policies driving the direction.[4]
- Run a workshop with others across the trust to justify the decision to be a learning organisation, and promoting a culture of lifelong learning.[4]
- Undertake a political, economic, sociological and technological (PEST) analysis to focus on factors external to your trust, and determine the drivers for your being a learning organisation.[4]

*Stage 5: Document your learning, competence, performance and standards of service delivery*

Keep the following:

- notes of reading and action plan for working through the practical tools[4]
- your updated PDP
- the training needs assessment of staff for whom you are responsible
- the completed PEST analysis
- notes of the workshop and organisational development plan.

---

**Box 6.7:**   Case study continued

Theresa continued to build on the momentum towards being a learning organisation in her post as education and training co-ordinator. The workshop she facilitated to create a strategy and statement of intent concluded with the setting of evaluation measures for the strategy of the effectiveness, outcomes and contributions to organisational objectives. Using this approach ensured that the trust board would be investing in and monitoring the evolution of the learning organisation culture.

---

# Example cycle of evidence 6.3

- Focus: teaching and training
- Other relevant focus: relationships with patients

---

**Box 6.8:**   Case study – teaching on the 'expert patient' programme

Steve is the primary care manager who is responsible for establishing and promoting the 'expert patient' programme. He has sent out flyers to GP practices, pharmacies and voluntary groups so that they can encourage patients with chronic conditions, who could benefit from learning self-help skills, to attend. This, together with the posters in libraries and other community settings and adverts in local papers, has resulted in a good response from patients. Steve wants to ensure the smooth running of the courses he is going to run.

---

This is just an example. Keep your task simple. You could choose three or four cycles of evidence to demonstrate your competence as a teacher each year.

*Stage 1: Select your aspirations for good practice*

The excellent healthcare teacher:

- arranges the delivery of education and training in a well-organised way that enables learning and accommodates other teachers' styles and learners' needs.

*Stage 2: Set the standards for your outcomes*

Outcomes might include:

- a tutorial plan
- mastery of a new skill as a teacher
- a teaching strategy that is implemented
- learner feedback
- evaluation of teaching programmes.

- Educational events are well organised in such a way as to enable the teachers to perform at their best and optimise learning.

*Stage 3A: Identify your learning needs*

- Keep a reflective diary: record your observations about organising educational events for all types of learners including lay people attending the 'expert patient' programme.[5] Include the ability to organise and operate audiovisual equipment, e.g. setting up PowerPoint presentations with a projector, the replacement of a bulb in an overhead projector, etc. Other parameters include producing handouts, finding a venue, the course administration, managing costs within budget, booking speakers, finalising a programme to suit the learning objectives and the nature of the audience, and advertising the meeting.
- Record any queries posed by participants on the course you are teaching or that you cannot answer (e.g. matters of fact or best practice, practical issues such as contact details), and plan to find out more information and respond to them after the event.
- Review of an audiotape or videotape of yourself conducting a session by a colleague or other trained 'expert' patient.

## Stage 3B: Identify your service needs

> Any of the needs assessment exercises in 3A may also reveal service needs.

- Obtain feedback from speakers or others with a role in organising the meeting using an anonymised evaluation form.
- Obtain feedback from participants at an educational event by using a specific evaluation form spanning the structure, process and outcome overall and of individual sessions.
- Compare the feedback from one course with another.

## Stage 4: Make and carry out a learning and action plan

- Ask a health promotion expert about the variety of approaches available for implementing different self-help strategies in order to educate patients as part of the 'expert patient' programme.
- Arrange tutorials from patients with a chronic condition relating to a clinical area of the 'expert patient' programme giving lay perspectives and describing points that need emphasis.

## Stage 5: Document your learning, competence, performance and standards of service delivery

- Continue your reflective diary once the 'expert patient' programme is in full swing. Record problems and requirements for the practical organisation of the programme and difficult to answer queries from participants on the programme.
- Keep notes from tutorials with patients of the key points learnt and how the plans for the programme are revised in response.
- Take notes at the meeting with the health promotion expert and record your reflections on further reading about educating patients undertaken as a result.
- Obtain feedback from speakers and facilitators involved with delivering the 'expert patient' programme.
- Obtain feedback from patients attending the 'expert patient' programme, with details of changes in behaviour at follow up if you are able to arrange that.

---

**Box 6.9:**   Case study continued

Steve was thrilled by the appreciation of those attending the course. The speakers and facilitators enjoyed themselves too. For many of them, it was the first time that they had taught patients in a group in a semi-formal way. Most of the speakers and facilitators had attended the session that Steve arranged for them to consider what pace, style of delivery and content would suit patients' needs and characteristics. That pre-course preparation really paid off according to the feedback from patients who attended the programme. Steve distributed questionnaires for patients attending to return by Freepost three months later to give further feedback of the benefits of attending the programme over time.

---

# References

1   Knowles MS (1984) *Androgogy in Action: applying modern principles of adult learning.* Jossey-Bass, San Francisco.

2   Pace CR (1963) College and university environmental scales. In: *Technical Manual.* Education Testing Service, Princeton, New Jersey.

3   Chambers R, Wakley G, Iqbal Z and Field S (2002) *Prescription for Learning: techniques, games and activities.* Radcliffe Medical Press, Oxford.

4   Garcarz W, Chambers R and Ellis S (2003) *Make your Healthcare Organisation a Learning Organisation.* Radcliffe Medical Press, Oxford.

5   Department of Health (2001) *The Expert Patient – a new approach to chronic disease management for the 21st century.* Department of Health, London.

# 7

# Giving feedback effectively

Constructive feedback is the art of holding conversations with learners about their performance and it has two elements; it should contain enough specific detail and advice to enable the recipient to reflect on and enhance their practice and it should be positive and supportive in tone.

Effective feedback has an impact not only on the teaching/learning processes but also gives messages to students about their effectiveness and worth. It has an indirect effect on their academic self-esteem.

Some healthcare teachers seem to struggle to give 'feedback with teeth', i.e. feedback containing enough specific examples of where a learner's performance needs to be improved (sometimes confusingly called negative feedback) without doing it in a 'negative' or unhelpful way. Indeed you often hear teachers say that in a situation where time is short, it is better just to concentrate on aspects the learner needs to improve, without seeming to realise that this and being encouraging in tone are not mutually exclusive.

## Constructive feedback

It is important that as well as being positive in tone (for reasons of the learner's self-esteem, morale and the development of good communication skills by observation of the teacher) we should aim to give feedback about both deficiencies and strengths. To see why this is important, consider the model of the development of expertise shown in Figure 7.1.

Starting in the top left hand quadrant in Figure 7.1 learners are blissfully unaware of their shortcomings until something happens to make them more aware. That might be the realisation when they start meeting patients that the education they had at university was not appropriate and that they are out of their depth. It could be a patient complaint or adverse incident or it could be feedback from a teacher.

This realisation is a painful process, often referred to as 'cognitive dissonance', but until we become aware we cannot start the process of learning. It is worth reminding learners that it's when you feel uncomfortable that you are just about to learn something. Too much discomfort however can be demotivating and some learners might give up at this stage if they feel that there is too

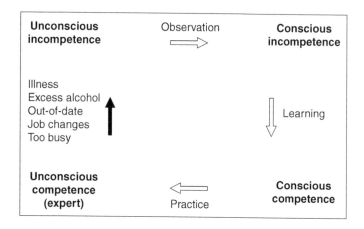

**Figure 7.1:**   Development of expertise (competency cycle).

much to learn or they will never be good enough. It becomes clear that some feedback about the other strengths they will undoubtedly have is supportive at this stage.

The process of learning, with all that that entails, can then proceed and we will master the new understanding, knowledge or task. We reach a stage where we know something new or know how to do something and can competently perform, so long as circumstances remain constant, represented by the bottom right quadrant of Figure 7.1. With practice and experience we then become expert, and we can apply and modify our knowledge and skills in new situations that we may never have met before. At this stage, in the bottom left quadrant, we could teach others. This is also the stage when through familiarity, we can lose sight of our strengths, as our skills become automatic. Feedback on performance at this stage needs to include things we are good at so that we do not accept them as commonplace, we reflect on them, keep them up to date and highlight them. In some ways, feedback needs to take us from left to right across the bottom of the competency cycle to make us aware of our expertise again so that we can effectively teach others.

It is possible to move back to unconscious incompetence from the position of expertise, in the direction of the shaded arrow, through a dementing illness for example, or degenerative disease without insight, or even failure to keep up to date. Feedback in this position is very likely to be difficult; this is another good reason to include a reminder of the learner's remaining skills and positive attributes.

This model provides a theoretical reason behind the observations that constructive feedback needs to contain commentary on strengths as well as things that need to be improved. It also reinforces the imperative for feedback to 'have teeth'. The skill of the effective teacher is, as always, to find the balance between support and challenge, and the best feedback is high on support and high on challenge. Figure 7.2 describes the qualities of feedback of different dimensions.[1]

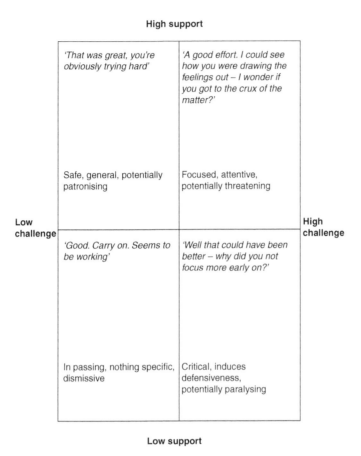

**High support**

| 'That was great, you're obviously trying hard' | 'A good effort. I could see how you were drawing the feelings out – I wonder if you got to the crux of the matter?' |
|---|---|
| Safe, general, potentially patronising | Focused, attentive, potentially threatening |
| 'Good. Carry on. Seems to be working' | 'Well that could have been better – why did you not focus more early on?' |
| In passing, nothing specific, dismissive | Critical, induces defensiveness, potentially paralysing |

**Low challenge** ... **High challenge**

**Low support**

**Figure 7.2:** Qualities of feedback.

# Four methods for giving feedback constructively

**Box 7.1:** General rules for giving feedback
- Focus on behaviour rather than interpretation.
- Give specific examples.
- Aim to be descriptive or sensory based rather then interpretive, non-sensory based.
- Aim to be non-judgemental rather than evaluative.

## Pendleton's model[2]

This model was first developed for use in giving feedback after watching video recording of consultations, but is useful as a set of general principles to be used in giving feedback after all sorts of activities, including practical skills, consultations, case presentations etc. It is a step-by-step model, in which each step is important, and is to be carried out in the order described below.

1  The learner goes first and performs the activity.
2  Questions are then allowed only on points of clarification of fact.
3  The learner then says what they thought was done well.
4  The teacher then says what they thought was done well.
5  The learner then says what was not done so well and could be improved upon.
6  The teacher then says what was not done so well.
7  Both discuss ideas for improvements in a helpful and constructive manner.

This model is useful for formal situations, with recipients who are not happy with feedback, e.g. the nervous, when the recipient lacks insight and to help learners say what is good about their performance.

## The SCOPME appraisal model[3]

In the Standing Committee of Postgraduate Medical and Dental Education (SCOPME) model, appraisal is used to mean what many in education call 'formative assessment'. This is about talking to learners and discussing their strengths and weaknesses in a helpful, constructive and non-threatening manner so that they can continue to work towards their learning objectives. The model is not as simple and clear-cut as some of the others presented here but nevertheless does follow the same sort of principles in order to give feedback constructively.

The SCOPME model has nine steps:

1  listen to the trainee
2  reflect back – for further clarification
3  support
4  counsel
5  treat information in confidence
6  inform – without censuring
7  judge constructively
8  identify educational needs
9  construct and negotiate achievable learning plans.

## The Chicago model[4]

This is similar to the other models but has the great advantage of starting with a reminder of the aims and objectives that the learner is supposed to be addressing. It has six steps as below:

1 review the aims and objectives of the job at the start
2 give interim feedback of a positive nature
3 ask the learner to give their own self-appraisal of their performance to you
4 give feedback focusing on behaviour rather than on personality (e.g. what actually happened, sticking to the facts not your opinions)
5 give specific examples to illustrate your views
6 suggest specific strategies for the learner to improve their performance.

## A six-step problem-solving model

This model aims to try to get agreement between two individuals for solving problems, agreeing goals, aims and objectives and so on. It depends on negotiations between two people who come to an agreement at two stages in the model.

It goes like this:

1 problem presented
2 problem discussed
3 problem agreed
4 solution proposed
5 solution discussed
6 solution agreed.

If you need to give feedback to someone whose behaviour is completely unacceptable, there are ways of delivering the information and still maintaining a relationship that will enable you to continue to work together and support that learner.

Consider these tips:

1 make sure the person is OK before you start
2 use a wake up, warning phrase
3 say very simply what is not right
4 give an example if necessary
5 relax the tone to allow for a positive response (usually an offer to improve ensues)
6 respond to the offer positively, but define specific measurable outcomes
7 do not be drawn into discussion on justification of behaviour or your right to judge
8 if your learner completely rejects your comments seek help, e.g. from your peers or line manager.

# Collecting data to demonstrate your learning, competence, performance and standards of service delivery

## Example cycle of evidence 7.1

- Focus: giving feedback effectively

---

**Box 7.2:**   Case study – learning to give constructive feedback

Bert is a consultant who has unsettled many a junior doctor by giving blunt feedback about their 'incompetence' when things go wrong. He finds it embarrassing to praise the good work of those juniors or nurse colleagues whom he rates highly. Having been sent on a course on teaching skills he wants to find out how he needs to improve his giving of feedback to others.

---

This is just an example. Keep your task simple. You could choose three or four cycles of evidence to demonstrate your competence as a teacher each year.

*Stage 1: Select your aspirations for good practice*

The excellent healthcare teacher:

- gives effective feedback, both praise and constructive criticism.[5]

*Stage 2: Set the standards for your outcomes*

---

Outcomes might include:

- a tutorial plan
- mastery of a new skill as a teacher
- a teaching strategy that is implemented
- learner feedback
- evaluation of teaching programmes.

---

- Be able to describe and compare at least two models of how to give feedback.
- Collect positive feedback from colleagues and/or learners about your usual feedback practice.

## Stage 3A: Identify your learning needs

- Obtain descriptive and specific feedback (written or oral, anonymised or identifiable) from learners or colleagues whom you have taught about the nature and quality and timeliness of your feedback.
- Keep a reflective diary: jot down your perceptions of how giving feedback went with a variety of types of people.
- Ask for peer review: giving feedback in trio work at a medical education course.

## Stage 3B: Identify your service needs

> Any of the needs assessment exercises in 3A may also reveal service needs.

- Organise a 360° feedback exercise from colleagues.
- Rate the extent of the time available for giving feedback to others in a training situation.

## Stage 4: Make and carry out a learning and action plan

- Attend a workshop on best practice in giving feedback as part of an on-going educational programme on teaching skills.
- Write an article about good practice in giving feedback for a local news-letter.
- Read an educational book and experiment with different models and approaches.

## Stage 5: Document your learning, competence, performance and standards of service delivery

- Obtain a written description of at least two models of giving of feedback, and reflect on which model works best for you and different types of learners or colleagues or situations.
- Keep anonymised copies of written feedback given to colleagues at their request for their own purpose, e.g. for their appraisal portfolio or to validate their competency in a clinical skill for instance.

- Record reflections on diverse ways you give feedback in any roles you hold, e.g. if you are a CPD or college tutor or appraiser.

---

**Box 7.3:**   Case study continued

Bert attended the workshop on giving effective feedback, and reflected on the variety of feedback he received from others about his own feedback skills. Over the course of a year, he was able to gradually improve how he gave constructive feedback to others and was consistently checking himself and trying to improve.

---

# Example cycle of evidence 7.2

- Focus: constructive feedback
- Other relevant focus: working with colleagues

---

**Box 7.4:**   Case study – using feedback to help others become consciously competent

As a teacher of undergraduates, Jed aims to help his students become consciously competent in taking a patient's clinical history by the time they leave their placement with him. When they arrive they are usually unaware of the gaps in their knowledge and skills about history taking in relation to the clinical speciality of neurology.

---

This is just an example. Keep your task simple. You could choose three or four cycles of evidence to demonstrate your competence as a teacher each year.

*Stage 1: Select your aspirations for good practice*

The excellent healthcare teacher is:

- able to give effective feedback to learners
- able to move unconsciously or consciously incompetent learners to conscious competence across a range of practice.

## Stage 2: Set the standards for your outcomes

Outcomes might include:

- a tutorial plan
- mastery of a new skill as a teacher
- a teaching strategy that is implemented
- learner feedback
- evaluation of teaching programmes.

- Be able to identify and reduce knowledge and skill gaps and any limiting attitudes of students and junior staff.

## Stage 3A: Identify your learning needs

- Develop self-recognition of your own perceived weaknesses in identifying the gaps in other people's knowledge and skill.
- Compare your rating of the competence of junior staff or students with that of teacher/trainer colleagues.
- Arrange for an audit of a student's performance by yourself, the student and another experienced colleague in a key clinical topic or non-clinical skill (e.g. record keeping). Compare your audit results and their interpretation, considering knowledge, skills and attitude.

## Stage 3B: Identify your service needs

Any of the needs assessment exercises in 3A may also reveal service needs.

- Consider adverse comments made about a student by patients or staff and your own role and responsibility as a teacher.
- Consider patient or staff feedback or comments about a student's behaviour and competence.
- Arrange 360° feedback from colleagues about your ability to motivate others in relation to learning and performance improvement.

## Stage 4: Make and carry out a learning and action plan

- Read about the Johari Window.[6] Discuss and reflect on the contents with colleagues.
- Go on a course in motivational skills.
- Undertake a postgraduate award in medical education.

*Stage 5: Document your learning, competence, performance and standards of service delivery*

- Review problem issues relating to competence using case studies with a teacher/trainer colleague.
- Record changes in knowledge, skills and behaviour of a student.
- Repeat one or more learning or service needs exercises described in sections 3A or 3B above and make comparison with the baseline.

---

**Box 7.5:** Case study continued

By the time the students leave their placement they have become consciously competent at history taking in relation to neurological conditions. They have their checklists of questions to progress through and are competent at probing further if the patient describes important symptoms.

---

# Example cycle of evidence 7.3

- Focus: giving feedback
- Other relevant focus: relationships with patients

---

**Box 7.6:** Case study – harnessing feedback from patients

The hospital trust decided that they had better invest some resources in harnessing patients' input into the teaching of junior medical and nursing staff. They ask the board member responsible for patient and public involvement to work with the hospital consultants to arrange for such patient input in their teaching.

---

This is just an example. Keep your task simple. You could choose three or four cycles of evidence to demonstrate your competence as a teacher each year.

## Stage 1: Select your aspirations for good practice

The excellent healthcare teacher:

- includes feedback from individual patients or patients' groups in setting the curriculum for students or juniors.

## Stage 2: Set the standards for your outcomes

Outcomes might include:

- a tutorial plan
- mastery of new skill as a teacher
- a teaching strategy that is implemented
- learner feedback
- evaluation of teaching programmes.

- Establish a patient panel with well-informed patients at the workplace, to advise about all aspects of teaching and training of juniors or students.

## Stage 3A: Identify your learning needs

- Ask patients for feedback on your own skills as a teacher; how did you do in explaining their condition and risks, etc. – were their expectations met?
- Give a slip of paper to patients to complete their views as they consult. Encourage comment on interpersonal skills.
- A patient might review a video of their consultation with you to give feedback on your teaching and explaining skills.
- Develop a patient satisfaction questionnaire using one that is relevant to a range of aspects of teaching and training, especially your skills and attitudes.

## Stage 3B: Identify your service needs

Any of the needs assessment exercises in 3A may also reveal service needs.

- An 'expert patient' might review a video of your tutorial with a student, junior staff, other staff member or another patient about a specific clinical condition (with their informed consent).
- Use a suggestions box or board at reception or in the waiting room for patients and carers to suggest ideas relevant to teaching and training.

- Obtain comments relayed from Patient Advice and Liaison Services (PALS) of the trust or from a focus group convened to explore problems or issues relating to training, e.g. information given out about the training of medical or nursing students.

## Stage 4: Make and carry out a learning and action plan

- Attend a workshop or course to learn more about possibilities and organisation of patient and public involvement and participation in teaching and what makes it more effective.
- Watch patients teach a student, junior or other staff member about a specific clinical area.
- Seek expert colleagues' advice about how students or junior staff gain maximum patient/carer input to their education while they follow the progress and concerns of patients with chronic or terminal disease over a period, within ethical guidelines.

## Stage 5: Document your learning, competence, performance and standards of service delivery

- Keep well-informed patients' commentaries on the standards of communication or clinical care by yourself and/or students or junior staff in the topic areas that teaching has covered.
- Use a technical measure, e.g. inhaler technique, to gauge the knowledge and skills of students or junior staff with respect to a clinical area after they have undertaken teaching of the patient.
- Keep a record of an event or activity for a patient group or population enabling their feedback into the education of students, junior staff or colleagues.

---

**Box 7.7:**   Case study continued

Everyone concerned is impressed with the insights that patients contribute to the way that junior doctors and nurses are taught and the clinical areas and skills that consultant teachers focus on. Subsequent patient satisfaction surveys improve as the way care is delivered becomes noticeably more patient-centred.

---

# References

1   Lambeth, Southwark and Lewisham Health Authority (2002) Out of hours project, accessed through www.trainer.org.uk.

2   Pendleton D, Schofield T, Tate P and Havelock P (1984) *The Consultation, an Approach to Teaching and Learning.* Oxford Medical Publications, Oxford.

3   Standing Committee of Postgraduate Medical and Dental Education (SCOPME) (1996) *Appraising Doctors and Dentists in Training.* SCOPME, London.

4   Brukner H, Altkorn DL, Cook S *et al.* (1999) Giving effective feedback to medical students: a workshop for faculty and house staff. *Medical Teacher.* **21**: 161–5.

5   King J (1999) Giving feedback. *British Medical Journal Career Focus.* **26 June**: 2–3.

6   Luft J (1970) *Group Processes: an introduction to group dynamics* (2e). National Press Books, Palo Alto, CA.

# 8

## Assessment

The term 'assessment' is used for the processes and instruments applied to measure the learner's achievements.

Assessment is a hurdle to be passed to allow progress to the next stage. This is 'pass' or 'fail', and is usually called 'summative' assessment by educationalists as it 'sums up' achievement at the end of a period of study. (This distinguishes it from 'formative' assessment that 'informs' you of achievements as you go along, highlighting progress and areas to develop while there is still time to do something about it. This can be known as 'appraisal' as we shall see in Chapter 9.)

Assessments are a statement to learners about what is important. If we say a subject will be assessed and make it a hurdle to pass to make progress, then trainees will study it, whether it is relevant or not! Assessments and course objectives therefore need to be aligned to help build towards the overall aims of the course.

## Link between aims and objectives and assessment

The first step in designing an assessment tool, then, is in curriculum development as you set your aims and objectives. In everyday language these words mean virtually the same thing, 'those things that we work towards', and are used interchangeably. But in education we make a distinction between them.

- *Aims* are broad statements of intent. For example, you might aim to produce a competent nurse or an effective healthcare teacher. They specify the broad direction in which you want your learner to go. They do not specify how far they have to go or how they will get there or how they will know when they are there.
- *Objectives* are outcome measures and are much more specific statements addressed at aspects of the aim. They are usually written in terms of what the learner will be able to do at the end of the course of study. For example, at the end of this post the nurse will be able to apply a dressing using a sterile technique, or by the end of this book the reader will know the

difference between aims and objectives and the relevance and purpose of each.

Certain words in objective setting are best avoided, such as 'to understand' – as it is much harder to demonstrate understanding and, although clearly necessary and not impossible, to devise an assessment tool to measure understanding. If you set a behavioural task in the objective such as to be able to list (recall), categorise (differentiate) and rank (prioritise) ... you are still testing learners' understanding but are also guiding them as to how to demonstrate it and giving yourself a marker to look for as you assess it.

# Domains of learning

Consider 'Bloom's taxonomy'.[1] He divided the three areas of learning into the 'cognitive' domain (pertaining to intellectual processes), the 'psychomotor' domain (processes of physical skills) and the 'affective' domain (attitudinal and emotional processes).[1,2] More simply this may be thought of as:

- knowledge
- skills
- attitudes.

A taxonomy is a hierarchical and orderly classification in which each level of competence builds on the one above (see Table 8.1).

**Table 8.1:**   Domains of learning

| | Domain | | |
| Level of competence | Knowledge | Skills | Attitudes |
| --- | --- | --- | --- |
| Base level | 1  Knowledge<br>2  Comprehension | 1  Observation<br>2  Imitation | 1  Receiving (listening)<br>2  Responding |
| Application | 3  Application | 3  Practising | 3  Valuing (advocating, defending) |
| Problem solving | 4  Analysis<br>5  Synthesis<br>6  Evaluation | 4  Mastering<br>5  Adapting | 4  Organisation<br>5  Characterisation (judging) |

Look a bit more closely at Bloom's taxonomy in Table 8.2 showing the cognitive domain (knowledge) with some illustrations of what skills might be demonstrated at each level of competence and some of the appropriate words we might incorporate into our objectives.[1] The right hand column will inform the development of assessment tools.

**Table 8.2:** Bloom's taxonomy

| Competence | Skills demonstrated | Objectives |
|---|---|---|
| 1  Knowledge | Observation and recall of information, mastery of subject matter | List, define, tell, describe, identify, show, label, collect, examine, tabulate, quote, name, who, when, where, etc. |
| 2  Comprehension | Understanding information: grasping meaning, translating knowledge into new context, interpreting facts, comparing, contrasting, ordering, grouping, inferring causes, predicting consequences | Summarise, describe, interpret, contrast, predict, associate, distinguish, estimate, differentiate, discuss, extend |
| 3  Application | Using information: using methods, concepts and theories in new situations, solving problems using required skills or knowledge | Apply, demonstrate, calculate, complete, illustrate, show, solve, examine, modify, relate, change, classify, experiment, discover |
| 4  Analysis | Seeing patterns, reorganisation of parts, recognition of hidden meanings, identification of components | Analyse, separate, order, explain, connect, classify, arrange, divide, compare, select, explain, infer |
| 5  Synthesis | Using old ideas to create new ones, generalising from given facts, relating knowledge from several areas, predicting, drawing conclusions | Combine, integrate, modify, rearrange, substitute, plan, create, design, invent, ask 'what if?', compose, formulate, prepare, generalise, rewrite |
| 6  Evaluation | Comparing and discriminating between ideas, assessing value of theories, giving presentations, making choices based on reasoned argument, verifying the value of evidence, recognising subjectivity | Assess, decide, rank, grade, test, measure, recommend, convince, select, judge, explain, discriminate, support, conclude, compare, summarise |

# Choosing assessment tools

Different assessments work better for different domains. For example, it will be less successful to assess practical resuscitation skills by asking learners to write an essay on the topic than to arrange a mock scenario.

# Knowledge

Information retention may be tested by a multiple-choice questionnaire (MCQ). Higher levels from comprehension to evaluation can be tested by extended matching questions, modified essay questions, scholarly essays, portfolio-based assessments and vivas. The latter however, although commonly used in higher professional assessments, are fraught with difficulties both in terms of reliability and validity.[3] Encouraging critical reflection and self-assessment might assist in developing learners through these higher levels just as much as working towards a summative assessment.

# Skills

The following tools all have a place in the assessment of learners' ability to demonstrate, show mastery of, or adapt, practical skills:

- *consultation/communication skills*: standardised patients, objective structured clinical examination (OSCE), teacher observation in daily work (video)
- *presentation skills*: audience feedback
- *clinical procedures*: OSCE, teacher observation, audit of case records, note keeping, letters and summaries
- *use of investigations or data handling*: audit of case notes, OSCE, teacher observation in daily work.

# Attitudes

Attitudes, beliefs and values are difficult to assess, but not impossible. A performance assessment would be most useful – knowing about something is not the same as carrying it out or believing it. This requires us to define ideal, acceptable and unacceptable behaviours.

To assess these attitudes we require information from those in a position to judge e.g. patients, senior colleagues and peers and possibly multidisciplinary colleagues. Bias can be minimised by ensuring that assessment is done by more than one person where possible. Criteria, standards and tools to enable us to judge need to be carefully developed.

# Assessments: desirable attributes

The 'ideal' assessment should be:

- *valid*: it measures what it is supposed to measure (if it has face validity as well, it also looks to the learner as though it is measuring what it purports to measure)
- *reliable*: it measures it with essentially the same result each time (learners with the same level of performance will be judged equally regardless of who administers it)
- *practicable*: it is easy to do in terms of cost, time and skills of the assessors
- *fair* to the learners and the teachers, e.g. differences between learners that are irrelevant to the subject being assessed do not affect the result, marking is not unnecessarily burdensome for teachers
- *useful* to the learners and the teachers e.g. it discriminates between good and poor candidates
- *acceptable*: in terms of, for example, cultural and gender issues
- *appropriate*: to what has been taught and learnt on the programme.

Sometimes there is a trade off between validity and reliability; increase in one is often at the expense of the other. Consider MCQ assessments for communication skills; they are very reliable, equally performing learners will score equally, but are likely to have low validity. The extent to which they can measure communication skills is low. At the other extreme we can increase validity by introducing simulated (or real) patients but reliability will fall off; we cannot be sure that learners of similar ability will score the same across all the simulated patients.

# Norm referencing and criterion referencing

Whichever tool we use, we need to make a judgement about how good is good enough i.e. what standard to apply. Norm-referenced tests rate a student's performance alongside others at that stage in the same cohort. Judgement is by comparison with each other. These tests give less of an accurate representation of what each student can do, cannot give useful feedback in terms of specific strengths and weaknesses and are not an encouragement for group learning – rather they encourage competition.

An example may be a test that the top 25% pass, whatever their score. Sometimes an individual mark is compared with the group average to rank students. These kind of tests may be used to control entry to the next stage in terms of numbers.

Criterion referencing rates students' performance to determine whether they have achieved mastery. Very often it is done as a form of formative assessment and it does not matter what their rank order is so long as they have achieved the competency. Clear behavioural objectives are required to define what the student should know or be able to do and standards of acceptable performance should be set.

# Collecting data to demonstrate your learning, competence, performance and standards of service delivery

## Example cycle of evidence 8.1

- Focus: assessment
- Other relevant focus: working with colleagues

---

**Box 8.1:**   Case study – assessing colleagues

Bob wants to learn to assess healthcare support workers undertaking their National Vocational Qualification (NVQ). As a nurse he is already familiar with assessing junior or student nurses and is unsure of the extent to which his expertise in assessing nurses can be generalised to assessing staff undertaking NVQs.

---

This is just an example. Keep your task simple. You could choose three or four cycles of evidence to demonstrate your competence as a teacher each year.

*Stage 1: Select your aspirations for good practice*

The excellent healthcare teacher:

- assists in making honest assessments of learners
- treats all learners equally and ensures that some groups are not favoured at the expense of others.

## Stage 2: Set the standards for your outcomes

Outcomes might include:

- a tutorial plan
- mastery of a new skill as a teacher
- a teaching strategy that is implemented
- learner feedback
- evaluation of teaching programmes.

- Be able to apply assessment tools appropriately.
- Understand the limitations of different types of assessment.

## Stage 3A: Identify your learning needs

- Carry out a significant event audit in relation to your role in assessment of learner and discuss it with peers with similar roles.
- Undertake a SWOT analysis of the assessment tools with which you are familiar and review their range and whether they are objective or subjective.
- Record your self-awareness of your own prejudices including those relating to other people's personality, their professional approach, age, background, etc.

## Stage 3B: Identify your service needs

Any of the needs assessment exercises in 3A may also reveal service needs.

- Discuss the weaknesses of any intended assessment methods with colleagues or with a course organiser.

## Stage 4: Make and carry out a learning and action plan

- Read up on different modes of assessment.
- Organise a tutorial with local educational lead or expert to learn how to overcome interpersonal difficulties relating to a learner. Recognise how your own personality attributes may interfere with the teacher/learner interaction.
- Learn to gather evidence on learners' performance from different sources – both positive and negative performance – to supplement formal assessments so that you can give regular formative feedback.

*Stage 5: Document your learning, competence, performance and standards of service delivery*

- Describe the curriculum for junior staff or a student, what assessments are undertaken and how the findings from the assessments are applied.
- Collect reports of the findings from the significant event audit and SWOT analysis undertaken in Stage 3A and the changes made in practice.
- Report how your teaching practice (content, style, time spent) has changed because of the assessments of previous learners.

---

**Box 8.2:**  Case study continued

Bob attends the assessor training course for NVQs. He meets assessors who also act as internal verifiers comparing standards in one workplace with those in another. He realises that much of his expertise as an assessor of nurse training can be generalised, but he needs to become more familiar and practised in the standards to expect of healthcare support workers.

---

# Example cycle of evidence 8.2

- Focus: teaching and training

---

**Box 8.3:**  Case study – complaints made against student or junior staff

Mary was fed up with hearing colleagues moaning about her GP registrar, Glen – his lack of punctuality, his brusqueness to patients, his refusal to take advice and his generally disrespectful attitude. Until now, Mary had made allowances for Glen as he was in the midst of a divorce and acting as a single parent to his three-year-old son. Today a patient has made a written complaint to one of Mary's partners, alleging that Glen had not diagnosed her skin cancer when she'd consulted him three weeks previously. She complained that he had barely glanced at her funny looking patch of skin then, and told her scornfully that 'she was letting her imagination run away with her', even though she had asked specifically to see a dermatologist. Now that one of the other GPs had referred her to the dermatologist, who had confirmed her worst fears, she wanted to lodge a complaint about Glen.

---

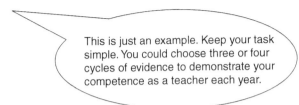

This is just an example. Keep your task simple. You could choose three or four cycles of evidence to demonstrate your competence as a teacher each year.

## Stage 1: Select your aspirations for good practice

The excellent healthcare teacher:

- ensures that patients are not put at risk when seeing students or doctors in training
- co-operates with any investigation arising from a complaint.

## Stage 2: Set the standards for your outcomes

Outcomes might include:

- a tutorial plan
- mastery of a new skill as a teacher
- a teaching strategy that is implemented
- learner feedback
- evaluation of teaching programmes.

- Ensure you have an established process for addressing complaints made about junior staff or students by patients or staff members.

## Stage 3A: Identify your learning needs

- Reflect on complaints made against junior staff or students by patients or staff and your own roles and responsibility as a teacher, line manager or health professional.
- Examine a significant event relevant to complaint.
- Undertake a patient satisfaction survey, or other mode of eliciting feedback, by patients about junior staff or students.

## Stage 3B: Identify your service needs

Any of the needs assessment exercises in 3A may also reveal service needs.

- Discuss, with colleagues and course organisers, methods and processes of handling complaints about students or junior staff.
- Compare your own current complaint processes with what others do or what is required by outside bodies (e.g. GMC, NMC, an accrediting body such as a university).

### Stage 4: Make and carry out a learning and action plan

- Learn about setting up effective complaints processes from professional regulation bodies such as the NMC or GMC, or from others with responsibility e.g. the deanery, university, PCO or medical defence organisation.
- Visit other teachers and trainers elsewhere to learn from their best practice in running complaints processes and minimising complaints.
- Role play problem issues and possible solutions in a trainers' group.

### Stage 5: Document your learning, competence, performance and standards of service delivery

- Report of a patient satisfaction survey including all doctors and nurses in the practice as well as the GP registrar.
- Record of a complaints process in relation to complaints or adverse comments made about junior staff or students, to include the way any identified deficits are fed back into the future educational programme.

---

**Box 8.4:**   Case study continued

The complaint is handled in a standard way according to the practice's complaint system. Glen meets the patient with the practice manager and you as GP trainer. Glen apologises for his manner and way he handled the consultation and the patient accepts his apology, so the case is closed. Mary arranges for the doctors and Glen to address the complaint as a significant event, and a plan is made for the responsible doctor to systematically collect and act on feedback from colleagues about Glen and future GP registrars or any students.

---

# Example cycle of evidence 8.3

- Focus: teaching and training

---

**Box 8.5:** Case study – being responsible for a junior who gives you cause for concern

You have a junior who concerns you. He worked in the same hospital speciality for 15 years before training with you. He has vast gaps in his knowledge and skills, but is socially adept. He refuses to accept that he needs to learn any more about his communication skills. A previous trainer has 'passed' him.

---

> This is just an example. Keep your task simple. You could choose three or four cycles of evidence to demonstrate your competence as a teacher each year.

## *Stage 1: Select your aspirations for good practice*

The excellent healthcare teacher:

- uses formative assessment to enable student to pass summative assessment
- assists in the honest assessments of learners.

## *Stage 2: Set the standards for your outcomes*

---

Outcomes might include:

- a tutorial plan
- mastery of a new skill as a teacher
- a teaching strategy that is implemented
- learner feedback
- evaluation of teaching programmes.

---

- Junior staff or student passes the summative assessment.
- Structural form is developed to collect everyday evidence of student's weaknesses.

## *Stage 3A: Identify your learning needs*

- Reflect on your own knowledge of different methods of formative assessment (e.g. using face-to-face or electronic media) and relevance of the usual methods in the light of previous students' feedback.
- Review the tutorial form and linked mode of formative feedback.
- Attend a lecture on patient input to education and discuss viability with others at a refreshment break.

## *Stage 3B: Identify your service needs*

Any of the needs assessment exercises in 3A may also reveal service needs.

- Compare your own students' pass rate in assessment with other pass rates elsewhere in the locality or in the region/country.
- Reflect on the relevance of usual methods for formative assessment in the light of previous students' feedback.

## *Stage 4: Make and carry out a learning and action plan*

- Attend an advanced trainers course.
- Conduct reading and reflection.
- Discuss the problems and solutions in a trainers' workshop.

## *Stage 5: Document your learning, competence, performance and standards of service delivery*

- Evaluation: pilot the revised form in your practice with colleagues – completed reports before and after a set period.
- Keep examples of formative assessment and students' responses (anonymised).
- Record the pass rate of the summative assessment.

---

**Box 8.6:**   Case study continued

You learn about different methods of assessment and you involve your junior in deciding what two methods might be most meaningful in determining his communication skills. You apply those methods and your junior has to face up to the findings, having planned the assessment with you and therefore 'owning' the results.

# References

1   Bloom BS (1956) *Taxonomy of Educational Objectives 1. Cognitive domain.* David McKay, New York.

2   Beard R and Hartley J (1984) *Teaching and Learning in Higher Education.* Paul Chapman Publishing Ltd, London.

3   Wakeford R (1999) Principles of Assessment. In: H Fry, S Ketteridge and S Marshall (eds) *Teaching and Learning in Higher Education.* Kogan Page, London.

# 9

## Appraisal

Appraisal (sometimes confusingly called 'formative assessment' by education-alists) has been defined as a two-way dialogue focusing on the personal, professional and educational needs of the appraisee with agreed outcomes.[1,2] By reflecting on practice, progress towards learning objectives can be gauged.

## Background to appraisal

As an educational concept, formative assessment has been around for a long time and extensively used for healthcare professionals in training.

Nurses have been engaged in portfolio demonstration of learning activity through their PREP (post-registration education and practice) requirements since 1995.[3] All community nurses – district nurses, health visitors and practice nurses – should be having appraisal or clinical supervision as part of that PREP process.

Senior house officers and specialist registrars have appraisal with educational supervisors, and general practice registrars undergo formative assessment firstly with the course organiser and then with their trainer when they are working in general practice. Non-principal GPs on the retainer scheme are offered an annual formative assessment with the local tutors. Those GPs in practice choosing to demonstrate their professional development through a PDP have been having peer appraisals with GP tutors for some years.

In addition, peer appraisal was introduced in *The NHS Plan* in 2000 and is now a contractual requirement for all doctors as a way of maintaining their personal and professional development.[4] Peer appraisal differs slightly from formative assessment, mainly in the nature of the relationship between ap-praiser and appraisee and the degree to which the appraiser is responsible for the overall progress of the appraisee.

One of the reasons appraisal seems to present a challenge for some health-care professionals is that it is also a familiar phrase from industry. The differ-ence there is that it is often used as a performance management tool and it is an uncomfortable mixture of development and judgement.

To make the confusion about terminology worse, the GMC has now linked the process of revalidation for doctors (clearly a summative process) to the appraisal process. Appraisal is an annual event and a cycle of five 'successful' appraisals for doctors is deemed acceptable for their revalidation, with clinical governance input.[5]

# Characteristics of appraisal

Some general principles of appraisal and how it is differentiated from assessment, with which it is often confused, are given in Table 9.1.

**Table 9.1:**   Characteristics of appraisal and assessment

| Feature | Appraisal | Assessment |
| --- | --- | --- |
| Prime purpose | Developmental 'informing progress' | Judging achievement 'summing up' |
| Participants | Appraiser and person being appraised | Learner and third party |
| Methods used | Structured conversation | Varied (*see* Chapter 8) |
| Areas covered | Educational, personal and professional development, career progress, employment (subject's agenda) | Learning objectives (third-party agenda) |
| Process informed by | Learners' self-assessment, day-to-day observation by teachers, other work-related inputs, results of assessments and examinations | Outcomes of standard, objective tests |
| Standards of achievement | Internal (personal to the individual being appraised) and negotiated with the appraiser | Predetermined by assessing body |
| Output of the process | Record of appraisal having taken place, agreed educational and personal development plan | Pass/fail |
| Confidential to the learner? | Yes, in most circumstances | No |
| Review/appeal | No need, as decisions should always be joint ones | Yes |
| Outcome | Enhanced educational, personal and professional development | Proceed to next stage |

# Carrying out appraisal

A good working definition of appraisal is 'providing a structured process by which the learner can be helped to define their own learning needs in the light of information they can gather or be given about progress from whatever source, allowing plans to be made to meet those needs'.

Here are some ideas of what you should be aiming for in the appraisal process with learners:

- the individual being appraised and the appraiser need to meet regularly. In the best schemes progress is reviewed frequently (some specify every 2, 3, 4 or 6 months). Annual reviews are insufficient
- nothing should come as a shock at a formal appraisal interview. Ongoing feedback all the time should make sure of that
- appraisal is not a substitute for day-to-day supervision, support and feedback on performance
- appraisers have an ongoing responsibility to ensure that the people whom they appraise can achieve the agreed objectives and, where necessary, give or direct them to help
- the individual being appraised plays the major part in setting his or her objectives but these must be set within the overall framework of what staff in that grade are expected to achieve or what learners at that stage are expected to be able to demonstrate
- self-assessment is an important part of appraisal but the appraiser must curb the tendency of the appraisee who may be unreasonably self-critical
- on the whole, appraisal interviews are best conducted on a one-to-one basis
- any promised level of confidentiality should be respected. The only exception to this is where aspects of poor performance come to light when the appraiser has a professional responsibility to protect patients. This proviso should be made explicit at the start of the process.

---

**Box 9.1:**   Skills for successful appraisal

- Listen
- Reflect back what is being said by the individual being appraised
- Support
- Counsel
- Treat information in confidence
- Inform without censuring
- Judge constructively
- Identify educational needs
- Construct and negotiate achievable plans

Listening is a key skill here. Remember what *listening* really means. It means keeping your mouth closed and your ears and brain open. It means not interrupting, not dominating the conversation, and not going in with prejudged ideas and conclusions already made. The balance of talking in an appraisal interview should be roughly 80:20 in favour of the person being appraised.

# Using appraisal to deal with problems

In the process of formative assessment of trainees you are likely to have to deal with problems from time to time. Sometimes these are problems brought to you by others, about the trainee. The trainee may not realise that there is a problem and when told may react angrily, deny the problem or accuse those making the comments of bias. There are ways around this and this section gives some advice on various techniques to try to help you in such a situation. However there are some learners who lack insight to such an extent that in these circumstances, if you are really struggling, others may be able to help you. Chapter 11 offers suggestions as to how to proceed then.

Even with peer appraisal you might want to address some difficult areas occasionally. It is less likely that you will feel able to tackle these however and you then, as an appraiser, have to make a decision. Are patients at risk and does the person being appraised lack insight? If the answer to both is yes, then you must stop the appraisal and start the poor performance procedure in your PCO or hospital trust. If patients are not at direct risk and/or the colleague has insight and is prepared to stop working in that area while seeking some retraining, it may be possible to work on and make notes of these issues. If your colleague becomes angry or defensive, the appraisal should be stopped and referred to the appropriate clinical governance lead. In peer appraisal there is no obligation, as there would be in an educational supervisory position, to deal with it any further.

---

**Box 9.2:**   Tips for dealing with difficulties

- *The whole process must be conducted using description not judgement.* For example:
  – description: 'You have not attended 50% of the training sessions and there have been three occasions when you were half an hour late for the start of the clinic.'
  – judgement: 'You seem to be lazy and disorganised.'
- *Keep it friendly.* Being descriptive allows you to assume the role of concerned friend and adviser rather than an outraged boss. Put aside any anger or aggression, both verbally and non-verbally, that you may feel. Show respect for the learner and they are more likely to show respect for you.
- *Identify and reinforce strengths.*

- *Problem areas need exact definition not generalisations.* For example say 'Your operations tend to take about 50% longer on average and your knot tying in the cases I helped you with was insecure and different each time' rather than 'You've got two left hands'.
- *Agreement will be much enhanced by objective evidence.* For example, witnessing of practical skills, team observation, written tests, review of notes or video.
- *Collaborate on constructive solutions.* Each specific problem area should have an agreed method of targeted training, the setting of objectives to be achieved and specified timescale.
- *Identify carrots and sticks to help ensure that the objectives will be achieved.* These need to be realistic: if something you promise to aid achievement is not delivered, this will seriously demotivate the learner. If threatened sanctions are not applied, future threats will be less effective.
- *Troubleshoot subsequent progress.* For instance, remove minor obstacles before they become major. Keep tabs on the situation – hoping of course to catch the learner doing things right. Review regularly until the learner is back on course.
- *Be unyielding in your minimum expectations.* If you have insisted that the trainee attends 70% of a training programme and they do not then comply, then you must keep to the sanction you put in place earlier.

# Collecting data to demonstrate your learning, competence, performance and standards of service delivery

## Example cycle of evidence 9.1

- Focus: appraisal

---

**Box 9.3:**   Case study – dealing with hostility from someone being appraised

Graham has cancelled his appraisal interview twice at short notice, but you both meet on the third booked date and time. He sent you his completed paperwork one week ago after you had rung to prompt him. What he has sent in is rather sketchy and the PDP has very little information and does not refer to learning undertaken as a result of last year's version of his PDP. As you start the interview, Graham appears to be hostile and silent.

---

## Stage 1: Select your aspirations for good practice
The excellent healthcare teacher:

- undertakes an honest and fair appraisal.

## Stage 2: Set the standards for your outcomes

Outcomes might include:

- a tutorial plan
- mastery of a new skill as a teacher
- a teaching strategy that is implemented
- learner feedback
- evaluation of teaching programmes.

- You need to understand and be able to explain the purpose of appraisal and personal development planning.
- You should be able to enable others to undertake and maintain a PDP.

## Stage 3A: Identify your learning needs

- You need informal feedback from Graham at the end of the appraisal and more formal feedback from Graham and others you have appraised, fed back via the PCO.
- You also need a peer review by a doctor or nurse CPD tutor about how you explain the purpose and methods of a PDP – captured by trio work, audiocassette taping, etc., with subject's informed consent.
- Conduct a significant event audit in relation to the two cancelled appraisal interview dates.

## Stage 3B: Identify your service needs

Any of the needs assessment exercises in 3A may also reveal service needs.

- Conduct reflections and discussion with other appraisers at appraiser support group run by PCO or deanery with self-realisation of your own strengths and weaknesses.
- Record the remarks in your own feedback from the PCO of the doctors appraised and compare it with other appraisers' feedback.

- Record the outcomes of pooling of information from practitioners' PDPs across the trust – looking at themes and patterns that are emerging.

## Stage 4: Make and carry out a learning and action plan

- Attend the ongoing local training and support meetings for GP appraisers.
- Attend a local workshop for medical and dental and other healthcare CPD tutors about personal development planning. Run a small group there about best practice.
- Represent general practice appraisal on the strategic working party of the trust that considers outcomes of PDPs and appraisal and the pooling of information about common themes to inform allocation of resources for education and training activities as well as service developments.
- Read up on worked examples of PDPs.[6–8]

## Stage 5: Document your learning, competence, performance and standards of service delivery

- Collect feedback on appraiser performance and your own reflections on that feedback.
- Keep a record of the peer review conclusions and subsequent action.
- Keep minutes of the significant event audit discussion with fellow appraisers and the subsequent action in general, and with Graham in particular.
- Keep notes of the strategic working party meetings and action plan.
- Keep the contents of the workshop on PDPs and flip chart notes emanating from the small group work.

---

**Box 9.4:**   Case study continued

Graham's initial hostility and fear melted away with your persistent encouragement. He had come expecting to be judged harshly for his lack of evidence of learning or progress in his PDP. When he found you adopted a helpful manner, he thawed and the evidence of his learning and striving to improve his performance was teased out. You showed Graham how to compose a PDP in a meaningful way and offered to put him in touch with the local CPD tutor. However Graham told you that he had already had an offer from one of his colleagues with a 'brilliant' PDP to work alongside her on both PDPs. You arrange to phone him again in two months' time to see how he's getting on.

---

# Example cycle of evidence 9.2

- Focus: appraisal

---

**Box 9.5:**   Case study – being appraised as a teacher

You have been an appraiser for a year, but next month it is your turn to be appraised by a colleague. You check over your portfolio carefully as you want to impress your colleague with how comprehensive and thorough a practitioner you are. You ensure that you include sufficient evidence in your portfolio to show that you are a competent appraiser who performs consistently well and that you have documented data about your teaching skills in your one day a week post in health informatics at the local university.

---

This is just an example. Keep your task simple. You could choose three or four cycles of evidence to demonstrate your competence as a teacher each year.

## *Stage 1: Select your aspirations for good practice*

The excellent healthcare appraiser and teacher:

- provides information that shows he/she is a competent appraiser/teacher in a speciality subject
- shows that he/she performs consistently well as an appraiser/teacher in a speciality subject.

## *Stage 2: Set the standards for your outcomes*

---

Outcomes might include:

- a tutorial plan
- mastery of a new skill as a teacher
- a teaching strategy that is implemented
- learner feedback
- evaluation of teaching programmes.

---

- Attain a good peer review by the appraiser of your portfolio who is enthusiastic about your documented work.
- Provide evidence of your learners' development in pursuing their health informatics course in relation to teaching by you.

## Stage 3A: Identify your learning needs

- Obtain a preview critique of your portfolio by a colleague or 'buddy' when you think it is complete, to identify any gaps.
- Check that all areas are covered within portfolio: educational, personal and professional development, career progress and key areas of work with both objective and subjective evidence of your competence and performance.
- Look at the parallel appraisal from the university management of your academic work and reflections on previous appraisal and achievements of last year's development plan for overlaps and gaps.

## Stage 3B: Identify your service needs

> Any of the needs assessment exercises in 3A may also reveal service needs.

- Record the input into the university examining body and personal feedback from the external examiner about the running of the health informatics course.
- Compare the curriculum taught in health informatics against current NHS requirements for health informatics, looking for gaps or disproportionate emphases in the content of the course.

## Stage 4: Make and carry out a learning and action plan

- Attend a local seminar for people preparing for appraisal on how to get the best out of your appraisal, purposely taking the subject's perspective even though you are an appraiser too.
- Attend an advanced skills course in an aspect of teaching to develop a particular interest or expertise.
- Plan and undertake educational research into an area of special interest that spans appraisal and teaching activities e.g. improving interpersonal skills, helping other people to change their behaviour, or enhancing multidisciplinary working.

*Stage 5: Document your learning, competence, performance and standards of service delivery*

- Keep your appraisal portfolio and appraiser's report with your agreed action plan.
- Keep the external examiner's report for the health informatics course including material relevant to your performance.
- Keep the appraisal of your performance as a teacher and outstanding training needs from colleague or line manager at university.
- Keep a certificate of attendance, accreditation or qualifications gained at the teaching skills course.

---

**Box 9.6:**   Case study continued

You looked forward to your appraisal as the day drew nearer as a chance to talk about your achievements to a colleague who was really interested in all that you had been doing. In the event, it was an even better session than you anticipated as your appraiser posed some challenging questions for you. You ended up talking about where your career was heading, and by the end of the appraisal, when the paperwork was completed, you left with a great deal to think through about your ongoing personal development and potential opportunities.

---

# Example cycle of evidence 9.3

- Focus: poor performance in others
- Other relevant focus: appraisal

---

**Box 9.7:**   Case study – separating out poor performance from appraisal

The date of your appraisal with Chris has been fixed for several months, being in the last month of her placement with you. You ask colleagues to complete a 360° feedback questionnaire about Chris because one or two have hinted that they will be glad to see Chris move on elsewhere – but you have been too busy until now to ask for any specific information. The only piece of evidence that you have of Chris' poor performance is a recent audit. This revealed that Chris had not acted upon two abnormal results sent back from the laboratory but had simply filed them in the patients' notes.

Soon after the appraisal discussion begins, Chris bursts into tears as she has already seen the 360° feedback report and knows what is coming. However, a brief discussion shows that she lacks insight and feels the staff were wrong to criticise her and they seem to pick on her unfairly. When challenged about the filing of the abnormal results, Chris declares that it is not attributable to her but the fault of the clerical staff who filed them away. You officially stop the appraisal as Chris is still tearful, but are not sure whether to reconvene another day when Chris has calmed down, or if you should be following the poor performance procedures (if you knew what they were).

---

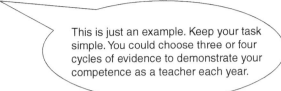

This is just an example. Keep your task simple. You could choose three or four cycles of evidence to demonstrate your competence as a teacher each year.

## Stage 1: Select your aspirations for good practice

The excellent healthcare teacher:

- undertakes an honest and fair appraisal
- ensures that patients are not put at risk by practitioners in training.

## Stage 2: Set the standards for your outcomes

Outcomes might include:

- a tutorial plan
- mastery of a new skill as a teacher
- a teaching strategy that is implemented
- learner feedback
- evaluation of teaching programmes.

- You should be able to recognise poor performance in a trainee for whom you are responsible at an early stage.
- You should be able to minimise or avoid harm to patients or NHS services from poor performance in a trainee or other learner.

## Stage 3A: Identify your learning needs

- Compare audits of the performance of the trainee with those of colleagues from the same discipline in the workplace.
- Obtain feedback from colleagues as to your listening skills when work had been left undone and they commented on the trainee's performance in an *ad hoc* way e.g. at coffee breaks.
- Read and reflect on methods of formative assessment and whether you know how to, and do, apply those methods to help the trainee understand what performance is expected.

## *Stage 3B: Identify your service needs*

Any of the needs assessment exercises in 3A may also reveal service needs.

- Phone the lead in the trust or local professional committee about procedures in place for addressing poor performance of clinicians, or the lead at the local training institution where the trainee is registered. Read through the current guidance and the steps you should take.
- Obtain copies of past reports of the trainee's performance, or if this is not possible, discuss your concerns with a previous trainer or person responsible for the trainee's qualifying programme.

## *Stage 4: Make and carry out a learning and action plan*

- Identifying your personal learning needs or service needs will have provided learning material.
- Read up about the poor performance procedures in other healthcare organisations – search their websites and that of the GMC or other regulatory bodies.
- Talk to other trainers to find out if they have had similar problems in the past and how they have confronted poor performance in a trainee, with positive outcomes.

## *Stage 5: Document your learning, competence, performance and standards of service delivery*

- Obtain documentation about the poor performance procedures that exist in your trust with an objective report about Chris and the stages you have embarked upon, the referrals made, the measures taken and the help planned.
- Keep a list of useful websites.
- Write a confidential account of Chris' poor performance and make notes of discussion with anyone to whom you have referred the case.

---

**Box 9.8:**   Case study continued

Chris did apologise the next day and explained that she has been distracted at work because of personal problems at home – which she realised she must sort out after the tearful session of the previous day. You arranged to discuss the 360° feedback and inappropriate response to abnormal results at an extraordinary tutorial the following week, but still carried on with your cycle of learning about poor performance procedures so that you could be prepared to address Chris' continuing poor performance if necessary.

---

# References

1    Standing Committee on Postgraduate Medical and Dental Education (1996) *Appraising Doctors and Dentists in Training.* Standing Committee of Postgraduate Medical and Dental Education, London.

2    Department of Health (2002) *NHS Appraisal. Appraisal for general practitioners working in the NHS.* Department of Health, London. Downloadable from www.doh.gov.uk/gpappraisal.

3    Nursing and Midwifery Council (2002) *The PREP Handbook.* Nursing and Midwifery Council, London.

4    Department of Health (2000) *The NHS Plan: a plan for investment, a plan for reform.* Department of Health, London.

5    General Medical Council (2003) *A Licence to Practise and Revalidation.* General Medical Council, London.

6    Wakley G, Chambers R and Field S (2000) *Continuing Professional Development in Primary Care: making it happen.* Radcliffe Medical Press, Oxford.

7    Chambers R, Stead J and Wakley G (2001) *Diabetes Matters in Primary Care.* Radcliffe Medical Press, Oxford.

8    Wakley G, Chambers R and Iqbal Z (2001) *Cardiovascular Disease Matters in Primary Care.* Radcliffe Medical Press, Oxford.

# 10

# Evaluation

Educational evaluation is a systematic approach to collection, analysis and interpretation of information about any aspect of conceptualisation, design, implementation and utility of educational programmes. Evaluation measures the teaching. It is not the same as measuring what students have learnt; that is assessment. Results of assessment processes however can be incorporated into evaluations, as in Figure 10.1.

Evaluation can concentrate on the effectiveness of a completed programme, when it is sometimes called 'product' or 'summative' evaluation and often carried out by independent observers. Or we can look at programme quality, usually during the earlier stages and this is sometimes called 'process' or 'formative' evaluation. This is often carried out by development personnel within the department.

Elements of evaluation can be carried out by:

- learners
- teachers
- a third party.

## The evaluation cycle[1]

Evaluation is a vital component of the educational process. Like any monitoring process it is iterative. Without it curricula cannot evolve and develop in response to changing needs, resource allocation cannot be decided, and the professional development of teachers is more difficult. When we apply it to courses and study days, we often want to find out 'how the teacher did'. When we apply it to courses we often want to know, 'are we doing what we set out to do?'.

Kirkpatrick has described a hierarchy of evaluation, or four levels on which to focus our questions, and these have recently been adapted for use in health education.[2,3] Table 10.1 considers the four levels that apply throughout the whole range of evaluative techniques and situations.

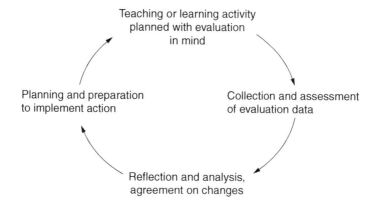

**Figure 10.1:**   The evaluation cycle.

**Table 10.1:**   Evaluating educational activities – the four levels[3]

| Level | Evaluation of: | Measure | Participant |
|-------|----------------|---------|-------------|
| 1 | Reaction | Satisfaction or happiness | What is the participant's response to the programme? |
| 2 | Learning | Knowledge or skills acquired Modification of attitudes or perceptions | What did the participant learn? |
| 3 | Behaviour | Transfer of learning to workplace | Did the participant's learning affect their behaviour? |
| 4 | Results | Transfer or impact on society | Did changes in the participant's behaviour affect their organisation? Were any benefits or problems noted as a result of these changes? |

# Participant evaluation

The commonest and quickest form of evaluation is to ask for participant feedback. We are all used to the evaluation forms given out at the end of a study day 'to help the organisers as they prepare for the next study day'.

Usual questions on such forms include: 'did today meet your expectations?', 'what aspects went well or did not go well?', 'what helped learning to occur or got in the way of learning?'. We can now see that these are level 1 evaluative questions in the Kirkpatrick hierarchy as in 'Reaction' in the top row of Table 10.1.

Sometimes the form will continue: 'what three things did you learn on this course?', 'what do you know now that you didn't know before?'; these are level 2 questions.

It is not common to be asked level 3 or 4 questions such as 'what things have you changed at work as a result of this course?' and 'what has been the impact of changes you have made?'. Clearly this is because these are delayed outcomes that cannot be evaluated on the day.

## What topics might you ask the learner to evaluate?

Evaluative questions for participants can also be designed around the stages of the educational cycle shown in Box 10.1.

---

**Box 10.1:**   Stages of the educational cycle

1   *Needs assessment*: Was the course relevant to you, were needs met or what was the extent of needs that were not met? Were problems solved or what was the extent of problems still remaining? Or were problems not tackled?
2   *Objectives setting*: Were the objectives clear? What important things were learnt? What else did you need to know about?
3   *Methods*: Were the methods appropriate: for example, lectures, group work, presentations, practicals and so on? Obtain learners' views of lecturers and group facilitators: could you read the slides and overheads in presentations; was there time for discussions and asking questions; how were the handouts?
4   *Assessment*: What three things have you learnt today? What was the 'take home' message?

---

Sadly, the opportunity to develop further after obtaining learner evaluation is sometimes limited by the questions (or responses) at the level of other issues – food, timetables, communications, sound, documentation, ambience and car parking. Sometimes the quality of the feedback reflects the level of insight the learners have into what a good educational experience would look or feel like for them, the degree to which they are confident about making judgements about their teachers, or some misunderstanding about the purpose of the questioning and how it will affect them. Sometimes however it is more to do with the quality of the questions and the level at which they are pitched.

## Remember that you do not have to evaluate everything!

Sometimes you see evaluation forms that have attempted to evaluate every single thing in a course with a very detailed questionnaire of several pages in length and complex marking scales to be completed. This is rarely necessary. You want to find out about things you can change. After a while of using the same form you will want to go back and consider the type and amount of useful information you are getting and whether the questions need to be pruned or altered.

---

**Box 10.2:**   Characteristics of a good evaluation tool

Characteristics of a good evaluation include being:

- appropriate: relevant to the educational programme
- intelligible: can be understood clearly
- unambiguous: means the same thing to all
- unbiased: does not trigger one response selectively
- simple: one idea only per question
- ethical
- pitched at higher levels on the Kirkpatrick hierarchy.[2]

---

An evaluation should be valid, reliable, simple, and practical, and probably anonymous. It can be quantitative (numbers) or qualitative (descriptive) or both.[4,5]

# Peer review

Evaluation by others not involved as learners in the teaching process is an important way to make revisions and modifications to our programme but also enables us to determine effectiveness, increase accountability and assist in decision making.

We might ask someone to evaluate us as course leader/instructor, the whole programme, the form of instruction, the technology, the environment, support services, levels of use, cost, outcomes, management, curriculum materials or impact on learners. Each type of investigation will require different methods and each will tell us more or less about the essential features of our teaching.

## Teaching evaluation

Peer review of the teaching process itself, having a colleague sit in and observe us as we teach, is a cornerstone of quality control in teaching institutions. As a method of personal and professional development for teachers it is a powerful tool. In addition it can be a useful way to evaluate the effectiveness of a course or even a department.

How to measure the teaching under observation however and make judgements about efficacy are not easy tasks. We need to know what makes teaching effective (what criteria matter), how to discriminate between good and excellent practitioners (what standards to apply) and how to spot it happening (what tools are needed).

You might consider asking a colleague to observe your next teaching session and ask them for their comments on what they saw. Similarly you could get used to the idea of critiquing your teaching by videoing yourself and doing a self-evaluation first. It would be an effective way of demonstrating your commitment to professional development in your personal learning plan.

# External evaluators

There are several methods of third-party programme evaluation.

## Objectives approach

This method looks for consistency or 'alignment' between goals, experiences, and outcomes using a pre-test, post-test design. Behaviours can be measured either by norm-referenced or criterion-referenced tests. It measures student progress against course aims.

## Goal-free approach

In this method the external evaluator is unaware of the stated goals and objectives of the course. The process determines value and worth of the programme based on outcomes or the effects and quality of those effects, whether intended or not. This has the advantage of revealing hidden strengths of a course to its developers but cannot answer the question 'are we doing what we set out to do?'.

## 'CIPP' approach

This is based on the explicit premise that evaluation is a tool to help make programmes better. Through it, information is collected from a variety of sources to provide a basis for making better decisions. It consists of four phases looking at different aspects:

- Context
- Input

- **Process**
- **Product.**

## Naturalistic approach

Here we have a model that takes into account participants' definitions of key concerns and issues. The mode of data collection is qualitative. It allows the learners to set the investigative agenda and determine the criteria for evaluation. Throughout, the language that is used and the mode of presenting the findings is intended to be accessible to participants.

The timing of the evaluation of educational activities in relation to the activity is an important area to be considered. Self-reported satisfaction with courses fades over time as participants return to work and find it hard to implement changes they may have learnt on the course. Good outcome scores in early evaluation may not therefore be sustained, or achieved, if evaluation is carried out too far from the event. But similarly, later less good performance in evaluation may give a better overall judgement about the impact of the course.

So, which aspects to measure, using which marker and when are integral to the success of an evaluation tool.

# Collecting data to demonstrate your learning, competence, performance and standards of service delivery

## Example cycle of evidence 10.1

- Focus: evaluation
- Other relevant foci: probity and research

---

**Box 10.3:**   Case study – evaluating your students' performance

Your colleague wishes to audit the effectiveness of different methods of education of the students who are placed with your practice or directorate. She invites you all to join in the study. She has adapted a research study published in a medical journal. On reading her plan you think that the feedback from patients who are evaluating the students' performance will mean that patients will not be receiving their usual NHS care and this is really an educational research study. The evaluation cannot be construed as an 'audit' as she had initially believed.

---

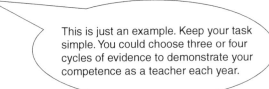

This is just an example. Keep your task simple. You could choose three or four cycles of evidence to demonstrate your competence as a teacher each year.

## Stage 1: Select your aspirations for good practice

The excellent healthcare teacher:

- protects patients' rights and makes sure that they are not disadvantaged by taking part in research
- evaluates the effectiveness of teaching.

## Stage 2: Set the standards for your outcomes

Outcomes might include:

- a tutorial plan
- mastery of a new skill as a teacher
- a teaching strategy that is implemented
- learner feedback
- evaluation of teaching programmes.

- Find established guidelines describing the limits of audit of clinical and non-clinical education and service provision so as to be sure what activities can be considered as audit and what research.
- Obtain approval of new research by local ethics committees within the research governance framework.
- Keep a log showing the monitoring of adherence of all research projects or initiatives to approved research protocols by the team.

## Stage 3A: Identify your learning needs

- Read through the frequently asked questions and answers on the Department of Health's website relating to research governance – consider if you are able to answer the questions before reading the answers.[6]
- Submit a revised audit plan to compare different ways of delivering education to students, adapted from the proposed research project, to the chair of the local research ethics committee to check that he/she agrees that the audit proposal does not fall within the definition of research.

- Discuss with local research lead how patient feedback can be sought in any form of evaluation without being construed as falling within the umbrella of research.
- Find out how others have used information from evaluation of modes of delivery of education to make improvements at operational or strategic levels.

## Stage 3B: Identify your service needs

> Any of the needs assessment exercises in 3A may also reveal service needs.

- Undertake a significant event audit in relation to a research study being undertaken by a healthcare colleague without prior approval being sought.
- Compile a list of ways that you or other teaching colleagues have undertaken evaluation of the delivery of education, in the last year. Get more information from those commissioning education about what evaluation they expect to be undertaken and how they expect it to be carried out.

## Stage 4: Make and carry out a learning and action plan

- Obtain documents about research governance from the Department of Health's website,[6] or your PCO, and read through them. Find out what measures the practice should be taking in order to comply with research governance when involving practice patients in research.
- Study the application form for local ethical approval of a research study, to be able to understand the limits on obtaining patients' views as part of audit of delivery of education or clinical and service management.
- Undertake a short tutorial from the local clinical governance lead about good practice in obtaining patients' views through audit, research and patient involvement activities. Include good practice in informed consent as recommended by the Department of Health or trust.[6]
- Work with the practice or trust manager to produce guidelines for anyone undertaking educational research.
- Set up a reporting and monitoring system in your practice for research being undertaken, if one does not already exist.

*Stage 5: Document your learning, competence, performance and standards of service delivery*

- Document a comparison of your own practice with answers to the frequently asked questions on the Department of Health's website about research governance.[6]
- Keep the response letter from the chair of the local research ethics committee about the query and the subsequent revised audit plan to ensure that work does not fall within the definition of research.
- File a copy of the practice guidelines for those contemplating research projects.
- Keep a copy of the guidance on research governance, with a page of reflection about how it applies to your own practice and trust.
- Make a list of the types of evaluation used by teaching colleagues, and reflections on their strengths and weaknesses.

---

**Box 10.4:** Case study continued

Now that your colleague has a clearer idea of what constitutes audit and what research, she obtains and submits the paperwork for ethics committee approval for a research study comparing different methods of delivering education to students. She is convinced that patient feedback is an important facet of the evaluation she plans, as well as the input by learners and teachers. The patients concerned on this occasion are a vulnerable group with varying complexity of mental health problems, so the chair of the ethics committee requests an ethical application as the evaluation involves some teachers interviewing patients to obtain their views.

---

# Example cycle of evidence 10.2

- Focus: evaluation

---

**Box 10.5:** Case study – using Kirkpatrick's hierarchy for evaluation[2]

Jake is starting out as a teacher having been newly appointed as a very part-time lecturer alongside his clinical work. He believes that evaluation is important and wants to do it correctly. He wants to learn how to undertake evaluation that encompasses the higher stages of the Kirkpatrick hierarchy (*see* page 148).[2]

---

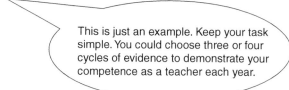

This is just an example. Keep your task simple. You could choose three or four cycles of evidence to demonstrate your competence as a teacher each year.

## Stage 1: Select your aspirations for good practice

The excellent healthcare teacher:

- ensures that evaluation of his/her teaching and the learning by students is meaningful.

## Stage 2: Set the standards for your outcomes

Outcomes might include:

- a tutorial plan
- mastery of a new skill as a teacher
- a teaching strategy that is implemented
- learner feedback
- evaluation of teaching programmes.

- Evaluation of teaching and learning addresses at least the first three levels of the Kirkpatrick hierarchy.[2]

## Stage 3A: Identify your learning needs

- Self-assess the last three forms of evaluation you have used. To what extent do each address:
  - satisfaction or happiness
  - knowledge or skills acquired or modifications of attitudes or perceptions
  - transfer of learning to workplace
  - transfer or impact on society?
- Write out one or two questions for use as an evaluation questionnaire and ask a group of teaching or training colleagues to comment on the questions as to their fit with the end points of learning in the previous exercise.

## Stage 3B: Identify your service needs

> Any of the needs assessment exercises in 3A may also reveal service needs.

- Organise a SWOT analysis of all the evaluation forms used for education and training or development that you and colleagues can collect, compared against the levels of the Kirkpatrick hierarchy.[2] Determine which evaluation forms already exist that measure knowledge and skills acquired, the modification of attitudes or perspectives, or the transfer of learning to the workplace or beyond, and can be classed as meaningful.
- Look for an opportunity to determine if evaluation techniques that you or other teachers have used can gauge outputs of learning. Ask a patient panel or individual patients if they think that what is being evaluated is important to patients, or compare what is being measured with what is known about patients' priorities in the delivery of healthcare.[2]

## Stage 4: Make and carry out a learning and action plan

- Read the original material written by Kirkpatrick[2] and authors reporting patients' priorities in relation to healthcare[7,8] and reflect on implications for your practice of evaluation and your own situation as a teacher (e.g. the extent to which what students learn is directly linked to their everyday job).
- Undertaking the personal learning needs analysis and trying to identify any service needs will provide a great deal of learning about the purpose of evaluation and the usefulness about what is being measured.
- Discuss with colleagues who have experience how to invite and utilise patients' views about evaluation or their priorities in provision of healthcare.

## Stage 5: Document your learning, competence, performance and standards of service delivery

- Keep the preferred evaluation forms capturing the extent and degree of application of learning – linked to the first three levels of Kirkpatrick's hierarchy.[2]
- Keep copies of the original literature[2,9,10] and your reflections about implementing the content in your teaching practice or approach to evaluation.
- Conduct a peer review of your preferred evaluation form and whether it is appropriate, intelligible, unambiguous, unbiased, simple, ethical and angled at higher levels of the Kirkpatrick hierarchy.

---

**Box 10.6:**   Case study continued

Jake learns a great deal about the Kirkpatrick hierarchy and produces evaluation forms that link to the four levels of the hierarchy.[2] He asks for evidence or examples of how students' learning will be applied in practice, so that the participants on his courses welcome the opportunity to give feedback as it helps them to consolidate what they have learnt from his session.

---

# Example cycle of evidence 10.3

- Focus: evaluation
- Other relevant focus: record keeping

---

**Box 10.7:**   Case study – record keeping of evaluation

Tim works as an allied health professional and is also a part-time senior lecturer based at a university. He is an award leader and teaches multidisciplinary groups of healthcare students on a variety of postgraduate awards. He prides himself on keeping good records of his teaching and all the associated university processes from the validation of the award, to the planning and delivery of programmes, and evaluation of learning and the student experience. His attention to detail in record keeping comes in handy as he prepares for the evaluation of his university department's teaching by the Quality Assurance Agency's (QAA) subject review process.

---

This is just an example. Keep your task simple. You could choose three or four cycles of evidence to demonstrate your competence as a teacher each year.

*Stage 1: Select your aspirations for good practice*

The excellent healthcare teacher:

- records appropriate information about students and other learners, being able to provide information about learners' needs and performance in a manner, and at a time, commensurate with their educational role and responsibilities.

## Stage 2: Set the standards for your outcomes

> Outcomes might include:
>
> - a tutorial plan
> - mastery of a new skill as a teacher
> - a teaching strategy that is implemented
> - learner feedback
> - evaluation of teaching programmes.

- Obtain paperwork relating to students' and other learners' performance correctly completed and despatched on time to the relevant educational body or committee.
- Develop an understanding and knowledge of criteria and standards of effective evaluation of teaching in different circumstances.

## Stage 3A: Identify your learning needs

- Feed back report to yourself and the others in your team from the university committee or educational review about standards of record keeping of the course, overall, and individual teaching in particular. It should be accurate, comprehensive, and complete.
- Conduct a peer review of the teaching session.

## Stage 3B: Identify your service needs

> Any of the needs assessment exercises in 3A may also reveal service needs.

- Use the nominal group technique with teaching colleagues to discover and agree what changes are necessary to increase the effectiveness of record keeping.
- Undertake a significant event audit, for example of lost or incomplete records disadvantaging a student by preventing progress to next level.
- Undertake a comparative audit of completeness of records about any stage in the teaching process between teaching colleagues – and look how your performance at record keeping compares with that of your peers.

## *Stage 4: Make and carry out a learning and action plan*

- Meet with representatives from the educational committee or someone who has recently been through the QAA subject review or another external assessment, to go through the requirements for record keeping with other teaching colleagues.
- Read up about requirements for record keeping in university or other professional body's paperwork and regulations.

## *Stage 5: Document your learning, competence, performance and standards of service delivery*

- Record the results of audit of completion of records.
- Keep the report of the significant event audit and the subsequent changes in keeping of records.
- Document the minutes of the nominal group meeting.
- Keep a copy of the regulations about record keeping.
- File the report of an external review, e.g. that of the QAA.

---

**Box 10.8:**   Case study continued

Tim has very little additional work to do in preparing for the QAA subject review, as his records were complete and to hand. The department sails through the review process and scores a high mark. Tim and the other university departmental staff enjoy their meal out to celebrate.

---

# References

1   Wilkes M and Bligh J (1999) Evaluating educational interventions. *British Medical Journal.* **318**: 1269–72.

2   Kirkpatrick DL (1994) *Evaluating Training Programs: the four levels.* Berrett-Koehler Publishers, San Francisco.

3   Barr H, Freeth D and Hammick M (2000) *Evaluations of Interprofessional Education: a United Kingdom review of health and social care.* CAIPE/BERA, London.

4   Bowling A (1997) *Research Methods in Health. Investigating health and health services.* Open University Press, Milton Keynes.

5   Bramley P (1996) *Evaluating Training.* Institute of Personnel and Development, London.

6   www.doh.gov.uk/research/.

7   Wensing M, Jung HP, Mainz J *et al.* (1998) A systematic review of the literature on patient priorities for general practice care. Part 1: description of the research domain. *Social Science and Medicine.* **47 (10)**: 1573–88.

8   Medical Professionalism Project (2002) Medical professionalism in the new millennium: a physicians' charter. *Lancet.* **359**: 520–2.

9   Kirkpatrick DJ (1967) Evaluation of training. In: R Craig and J Bittel (eds) *Training and Development Handbook.* McGraw-Hill, New York.

10  Miller GE (1990) The assessment of clinical skills/competence/performance. *Academic Medicine: Journal of the Association of American Medical Colleges.* **65 (9)**: S63–67.

# 11

## The challenging trainee

Sometimes it all goes wrong. Sometimes the difficulty lies with the learner, sometimes with the teacher and sometimes the learner–teacher relationship. There are probably as many causes of inter-relationship problems as there are challenging trainees but there are some recurring themes to look at.

There are various ways that the trainer–trainee relationship may run into difficulties. These may include personal problems, underperformance, health-related issues (both physical and mental), stress, problems outside of medicine, such as family difficulties or illness, and disciplinary matters. Sometimes the problem is the post and the trainer, and not the trainee. It is obviously important to find this out. So get both sides of the story before jumping to conclusions.

Difficulties show themselves in many ways:

- non-attendance for teaching sessions
- non-participation in groups or destructive group behaviour
- not keeping up to date or preparing for the session
- failure in exams
- tardiness or failure to turn up for work
- incomplete tasks during work time, not answering their bleep
- problems with working in the team
- inability to take or give instructions to staff
- poor communication with, or complaints from, patients.

These are all symptoms of underlying difficulties and it can help to ask:

- what is the real problem?
- why has this happened now?
- what can we do about it?
- can we get back on course?

Just as in clinical practice, the treatment is less likely to work if the diagnosis is wrong. If the measures are aimed at symptoms, they may not address the real difficulty.

---

**Box 11.1:**   Common trainer–trainee problems

'The biggest trainer problem we find is lack of documentation.'

'The biggest and most difficult trainee problem is lack of insight.'

(David Wall, deputy postgraduate dean, West Midlands)

---

# The problems

A simple way to categorise such problems is to divide these into four main areas. These are as follows:

*   personal conduct
*   professional conduct
*   competence and performance issues
*   health and sickness issues.

Is there a problem? If there is, then the first step is to clarify things, to get both sides of the story, and not to jump to conclusions based only on one side of the story. Get onto the problem early. Do not leave it to the next appraisal or performance review. It may be necessary to investigate the problem formally, with written statements from the various individuals involved, and records of what has happened.

Many problems can be resolved at local level, rather than involve formal processes of a national body or regional organisation. However the principles of finding out the facts, using facts of the case and not opinions with constructive feedback and setting targets for improvement, and following these through, will hopefully work well in most cases.

The trainee will always have an employer. The employer may be the NHS trust, the university, or the general practice trainer in the case of GP registrars. Legally the employer must take the lead in all four areas of problems. Employers will have procedures laid down for discipline, performance and sickness issues. In the case of employed doctors, the trainee may approach the deanery for advice. What happens next will depend on the types and seriousness of problems encountered.

## Personal conduct issues

Examples of such problems include theft, fraud, assault on another member of staff, vandalism, rudeness, bullying, racial and sexual harassment, pornography downloading from a computer in the library, and attitude problems in relation to colleagues, other staff and patients. The trust (as the employer) will take the lead under its approved disciplinary procedures. The employer should inform the trainee at an early stage that he/she may approach their professional body or the deanery (in the case of doctors) for advice, particularly if there are concerns that any allegations are as a result of professional issues, and/or education and training difficulties.

---

**Box 11.2:** Code of practice for personal conduct issues

- The trust must follow an agreed disciplinary procedure.
- The trainee must be advised that they may be legally represented (by the British Medical Association or a solicitor, for example).
- National guidelines must be followed if a trainee is to be suspended.
- Pastoral support should be provided if needed.

---

# Professional conduct issues

Examples of such problems include research misconduct, failure to take consent properly, prescribing issues, improper relationships with patients, improper certification issues (such as the signing of cremation forms, sickness certification, passport forms), and breach of confidentiality. The trust (as the employer) will take the lead under its disciplinary procedures. In the case of doctors, the deanery will provide an input into such a disciplinary process via the clinical tutor, the GP trainer, the chair of the speciality training committee or the regional adviser (for specialist registrars). Any decision to involve the professional regulatory body is a very serious one for the health professional involved and, in the case of doctors, this will be a joint decision between the trust (or other employer) and the deanery. Approved procedures should be followed first at the local level, rather than reporting everything to the professional regulatory body at the earliest stage.

---

**Box 11.3:** Code of practice for professional conduct issues

- The trust must follow an agreed disciplinary procedure.
- The disciplinary process should include someone to represent the deanery (in the case of doctors).
- The trainee must be advised that they may be represented (by a solicitor, for example).
- National guidelines must be followed if a trainee is to be suspended.
- Pastoral support should be provided if needed.

---

# Competence and performance issues

Examples of such problems include a single serious mistake, or poor results clinically, possibly found as a result of audit, poor timekeeping, poor communication skills, poor consultation skills and repeated failure to attend educational events.

Hopefully most of these may be dealt with through the educational framework. The trust or other employer will need to take a lead in some of these problems, if there may have been a complaint from patients or relatives, and the possibility of a legal action. In the West Midlands there are mechanisms for further expert assessment and remedial training of doctors in such areas of communication and consultation skills, using the interactive skills unit.

An isolated serious mistake may happen to any of us and usually does not reflect the overall competence of the health professional concerned. If we are honest, many of us have been in this situation at some time in our careers. Such a mistake may lead to a formal inquiry. Pastoral support must be offered as such an event is highly stressful for all concerned. If the health professional learner's performance is consistently poor, even though all educational measures have been tried to put things right, then it may on occasions be necessary to inform the professional regulatory body. Obviously this is not a decision to be taken lightly, or on the spur of the moment. Such a referral may have momentous and unpredictable consequences for the health professional concerned.

# Health and sickness issues

Every doctor or other health professional must be encouraged to register with a local general medical practitioner, and consult with their doctor in the first instance when ill.

Ill health and sickness absence should be managed through the trust's sickness procedures and may include their occupational health service. It is not possible to give a generalised rule about the length of sickness absence, as each case needs to be considered on its merits. Where sickness absence does give cause for concern, then the views of a consultant physician in occupational medicine are essential in such cases.

There are guidelines on serious infectious diseases and other health issues, including physical and mental illness that may affect the safety of patients. These need to be consulted, and the advice of a consultant physician in occupational medicine is essential in such cases. Some areas have an independent confidential counselling service as well as occupational health services available to staff.

Sometimes a ruling is needed on time off for sickness before it starts to affect the date when training is deemed to have finished. For example, the West Midlands Deanery guidelines for the periods of grace before completion of training date may be affected are:

- three weeks in a four-month post, four weeks in a six-month post or a total of four weeks overall in the year for pre-registration house officers
- four weeks in a two-year period for senior house officers
- two weeks in a 12-month post for GP registrars.

# Transfer of education and training information from trust to trust

Health professionals may work for several employers throughout their postgraduate training, as they go through different jobs in a rotation, and progress through the different training grades. Sometimes a problem arises towards the end of a clinical placement in a particular trust. In such circumstances, remedial action may be put in place to remedy poor performance or other issues. In such events, the educational supervisor in the next placement needs to know about all this, to ensure that the remedial training continues, and assessments of successful progress are made.

We suggest that there is a transfer of information to the new educational supervisor on strengths and areas for further development (as identified by the outgoing educational supervisor). This is normally part of the health professional's personal learning plan.

# Prevention is better than cure

In all cases, regular day-to-day feedback on work is one of the best ways to learn. Constructive feedback works best. Regular appraisal and assessments are essential (as in Appendix 1). Collect information prospectively, especially about the health professional learner's adherence to agreed and accepted processes, such as the use of guidelines, furthering their own education, attendance at protected teaching sessions, contribution to research and development activities, audit, awareness of their own clinical outcomes and so on.

There is nothing worse than running into problems which, when we look closely at the situation, have been going on for some time, and there is nothing written down. The health professional in difficulty may then claim that they were completely unaware of any problem, and if they had been, they would have done something about it.

One of the keys to preventing or dealing with difficulties lies in the educational rapport between the learner and the teacher. The Johari Window, shown in Figure 11.1, is a model for thinking about communication.[1]

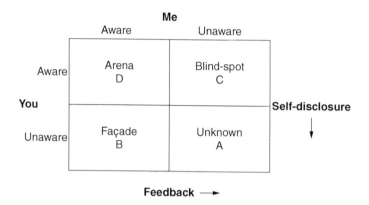

**Figure 11.1:**   The Johari Window.

The window represents how relationships are built up by an accumulation of information from 'self' and 'others' – me and you.

As we try to build relationships with our learners and trainees to increase the effectiveness of our teaching, this model might help explain why some people are considered to have communication difficulties or are labelled poor communicators, or worse still why some relationships become dysfunctional. Up to a point, the larger the arena, the more productive is the relationship.

To enhance relationships we need not change ourselves, but address the balance of these two basic behaviours of feedback and exposure or self-disclosure.

# Type A: little exposure, little feedback seeking

These people are often perceived as being withdrawn, aloof or impersonal, where the unknown square is the largest. This may induce resentment in others who may take the behaviour personally.

# Type B: increased feedback seeking, little exposure

These people decrease the information about themselves that is available to others, while requiring more from others, either through fear or a wish for power or control. Others may react by withdrawing trust or becoming hostile.

# Type C: increased exposure, neglect of feedback

These people are oblivious to the impact they have on others. They have a large blind-spot as the opportunity for feedback is rare. They may be confident of their own opinions and insensitive, with little concern for the feelings of others. Listeners may become angry and reluctant to tell them anything.

# Type D: balanced

These people have a large arena as feedback seeking and exposure are well used. They are open and candid. Initially others may be put on the defensive but when they are seen as genuine, productive relationships can follow. They induce an open balanced response in others.

Teachers and learners need to be sensitive about the covert content of the blind-spot, the façade and the hidden area and respect privacy about information kept hidden for reasons of social training or custom.

---

**Box 11.4:**   General principles that may help when addressing concerns about learners

- *Do it now*: tackle the problem when it occurs and not at the end of the placement.
- *Find out the facts*: do not jump to conclusions.
- *Explain the problem*: explore the issues with the learner, ask for their views or comments and plan how to get back on course.
- *Give support* and encouragement.
- *Document what you do*: appraisals, assessments, comments from others, incidents etc. and keep copies of all paperwork. Use the correct framework as laid down by your speciality training committee or Royal College or professional organisation.
- *Share the problem*: do not try to do it all on your own but get advice from others – other teachers, educational supervisors, your speciality tutor, your clinical tutor, your own line manager, the training programme director, the chair of your speciality training committee or the postgraduate dean's office.
- *Inform* senior colleagues as appropriate.

Having explored the issue, ask yourself:

- is this an educational issue that the learner and I can tackle between us with the tools available to us?
- is this a relationship problem or personality clash between the learner and me?
- do I need help from someone else to help guide this learner?
- does the learner need careers advice?
- does the learner (or teacher) have other problems such as physical or mental illness?

---

# If you think it's possible to get back on track

The next section covers a few techniques that might help, if you consider that the situation is retrievable.

## Is it a problem with the learner's stage of self-direction?

Try asking yourself:

* have I got a *dependent learner* – do they request coaching and guidance? Are they happiest with lectures from experts and extensive handouts? Do they seem to ask frequently 'Is this in the exam', are they keen to find out from you the 'right answer'?
* have I got an *interested learner* – will they engage in guided discussion, can they participate in goal setting and learning strategies, do they sometimes ask you what books to read?
* have I got an *involved learner* – do they engage in discussions as an equal, can they run and participate in seminars, doing background work and preparation for the group? Can they work alone?
* have I got a *self-directed learner* – do they look to you as a supervisor of their work, someone who delegates tasks and can be consulted as need be? Do they have the study skills to analyse their own learning needs and devise a programme of study to address them?

## Is there a mismatch of learning styles?

Consider identifying learners' learning styles, or at least be aware of the variation and offer a range of educational activities.

## Is it the trainee or is it the trainer? Is it the job?

Sometimes we might move the trainee to another post in a different practice or hospital, to enable a fresh start to be made.

## Is the issue related to group work?

Probably the commonest teaching setting is a small group and all teachers at one time or another will have experienced difficulties with the reactions and interactions of some members of the group. Revise the theories of group dynamics and check the roles that your learners are playing in a group.

## Is it an issue of time management?

Sometimes learners have full, difficult lives and the best you can be is supportive. Otherwise try to offer them advice about priority setting, delegation, planning, organisation and not taking on too much.

# If it is not possible to get back on track

You may come to the conclusion, alone or in discussion with the learner, that the situation is beyond your joint capacity to solve. It might be that just transferring to another educational supervisor, intermitting from the course to return later or changing career direction is what is needed. Good teachers respond positively to these situations as it should not be taken as a sign of failure but rather one of maturity, to recognise the limitations of a situation and know how to go about addressing them.

## Does the trainee need to be referred to occupational health or a doctor?

Does the trainee (or trainer) have other problems such as stress, physical or mental illness etc.? It is important in all teaching relationships to recognise the explicit and implicit boundaries. This is especially important in the healthcare professions when it is easy to slip into the role of problem solver or care giver.

Try to recognise when you are acting as a health adviser. If this happens, ensure that your learners have a GP to consult and know how to signpost them to occupational health if need be. This makes sure that they get impartial advice and protects you from a charge that you colluded in an issue that may have put patients at risk. If a trainee is better off not being at work, you might not give the same advice as their own doctor who is not also their line manager, e.g. if they plead with you to continue at work because the exams are coming up.

## Does the trainee need to see a careers counsellor?

Does the trainee need careers advice? Are they in the wrong career? What if the trainee is coming to the conclusion that he is a 'square peg' in a 'round hole'? Or what if you have come to that conclusion and they cannot see it yet? What if the onset of a degenerative disease is limiting their career options? The advisory skills required in this area are specialised. Most people working in the healthcare professions have invested a lot in terms of time and commitment to getting where they are now. It may be the result of a lifelong career plan, and the thought of changing direction can be daunting.

You need to raise this with the trainee and seek their opinions. If they agree, consider putting them in touch with specialist career counsellors. For further details *see* Chapter 12.

## Is this a disciplinary matter?

Sometimes these can be the easiest issues to deal with if trainees are guilty of obvious breaches of the implicit code of conduct such as fraud, theft or violent behaviour. In clear and significant breaches, such as persistently being under the influence of alcohol at work, all professional groups have made it an obligation on members to protect the public from incompetent or dangerous practitioners, and part of being a professional is to be aware of that obligation to report such practitioners to our regulatory bodies.

On the whole, deciding whether to institute disciplinary proceedings is a difficult decision to take and one that most teachers should not be taking on their own. Always discuss such problems with colleagues, either formally or informally, to gain a second opinion or advice.

# In conclusion

Most learner–teacher relationships do not encounter any of the problems outlined in this chapter. You might go through your whole career as a trainer and only have a handful of challenging trainees. It is all the more important, then, to have identified in advance routes to take and sources and ideas for help, as they can be very stressful times for both the learner and trainer.

Increasingly, a more systematic and structured approach to medical and other health professional education and training is being put into place. Such initiatives include appraisals, 360° feedback, annual assessments, revalidation, clinical governance and a much greater emphasis on the quality of care to patients. Such a structured approach is now beginning to pick up, at an earlier stage, some doctors and other professionals as they begin to run into problems.

# Collecting data to demonstrate your learning, competence, performance and standards of service delivery

## Example cycle of evidence 11.1

- Focus: the challenging trainee
- Other relevant focus: communication skills

---

**Box 11.5:** Case study – confronting trainees who do not want to listen

Kate just does not appear willing to take instructions from you or others in the team. She has almost completed her physiotherapy training and is undertaking her last placement in the community. She often tells you how they do it in hospital and then proceeds in her own way citing some evidence you've never heard of to justify her clinical activities. She has a similar dismissive attitude to some older patients whom she believes are 'wasting my time with their aches and pains – what else can they expect from old age?'.

---

This is just an example. Keep your task simple. You could choose three or four cycles of evidence to demonstrate your competence as a teacher each year.

*Stage 1: Select your aspirations for good practice*

The excellent healthcare teacher:

- communicates well with patients, learners, and other colleagues
- has an effective system for communication within the team
- is an effective teacher however challenging the trainee
- ensures that students or others do not put patients at risk in training.

## Stage 2: Set the standards for your outcomes

Outcomes might include:

- a tutorial plan
- mastery of a new skill as a teacher
- a teaching strategy that is implemented
- learner feedback
- evaluation of teaching programmes.

- Develop effective communication skills between you the teacher and learners.
- Become able to confront a challenging trainee, whose behaviour changes as a result.

## Stage 3A: Identify your learning needs

- Ask for feedback from the trainee about the placement, including questions in feedback format that cover the structure and process of giving care as well as interpersonal matters between the trainee and you as teacher.
- Undertake an audit of your own work in at least one clinical area of care where the trainee has indicated that there is evidence for a different approach.
- Undertake a significant event audit of a recent example whereby the trainee has adopted their own clinical approach against your advice or instructions or without asking for guidance when you judge they should have done. Involve all the team.

## Stage 3B: Identify your service needs

Any of the needs assessment exercises in 3A may also reveal service needs.

- Organise 360° feedback about you and the trainee from others in the practice or department team, to discuss at a tutorial. It is more equitable to discuss others' opinions of both of you.
- Use a consulting style rating scale for you and trainee for ten consecutive patient consultations each, to discuss and compare findings.[2]
- Request help from your lead for trainee placements. Find out if this situation is typical for this trainee from their past placements, or if it is something particular to you and the community setting. Ask how others have dealt with it, and how the lead thinks you should address the issues.

## *Stage 4: Make and carry out a learning and action plan*

- Review and reflect on the literature about communicating well with learners, other colleagues and patients.
- Prepare for and run a tutorial on communication skills for the trainee and others in the practice or department, or other trainees on various placements.
- Organise older patients to input into the teaching session and give their perspectives about e.g. osteoarthritis, Parkinson's disease. You will learn a great deal as well.

## *Stage 5: Document your learning, competence, performance and standards of service delivery*

- Repeat the 360° survey at a later stage in the placement if there is time, focusing on communication skills.
- Obtain learners' ratings of your communication skills seminar.
- Conduct a self-assessment from rating of your consulting style for ten patients.
- Keep a record of the significant event audit and action plan. Describe the subsequent change (if any) in the trainee's attitude and clinical behaviour.

---

**Box 11.6:** Case study continued

Meeting the two older patients in the teaching session does have a considerable impact on Kate's attitude, hearing at first hand their experiences of attending the local rheumatologist and neurologist respectively and receiving physiotherapy at the hospital outpatient department over the years. She starts to respect their struggle to live independently and overcome their disabilities. The evidence you have derived from a literature search on best practice, in one of the approaches to clinical care that Kate has disputed, shows that there is no conclusive 'right' way. You both agree that each of your approaches are justified and develop a growing respect for each other.

---

# Example cycle of evidence 11.2

- Focus: teaching and training

---

**Box 11.7:**   Case study – helping the trainee who fails their assessment

Jayne has just failed to pass her specialist exams for the second time. You admire her ability as a clinician and are disappointed that she has not managed to pass the examination. You are not too surprised she failed as she had rarely turned up for teaching sessions and always had a convenient excuse. She is devastated and is talking of switching her career to a different speciality area where there is less competition for the relatively few consultant posts. Her proposal to give up medicine and run a bar in the Mediterranean did not sound too convincing though.

---

This is just an example. Keep your task simple. You could choose three or four cycles of evidence to demonstrate your competence as a teacher each year.

*Stage 1: Select your aspirations for good practice*

The excellent healthcare teacher:

- encourages and enables learners to achieve their potential.

*Stage 2: Set the standards for your outcomes*

---

Outcomes might include:

- a tutorial plan
- mastery of a new skill as a teacher
- a teaching strategy that is implemented
- learner feedback
- evaluation of teaching programmes.

---

- Learners you teach pass speciality examinations according to their potential ability.

## Stage 3A: Identify your learning needs

- Compare the pass rate of learners whom you have taught, in any speciality examinations or other external assessments, with other cohorts of learners.
- Look at the scope of the speciality examination and any relevant past examination papers and check them against the curriculum of your teaching and clinical relevance of areas that the trainee has experienced. Are there significant gaps?
- Discuss your usual approach to establishing a learner's training and development needs at their induction or at an initial meeting, and thereafter in their post, with a teaching colleague. Is your educational analysis sufficiently wide-ranging and objective?
- Discuss Jayne's failure to pass the speciality examinations with her once she is over the initial shock of disappointment. Ask her if you can help more or who else could be recruited to tutor her, or give her more experience. Encourage Jayne to obtain feedback about her examination performance, if it is available on request, and talk through the reasons for any weaknesses and how they might be redressed.

## Stage 3B: Identify your service needs

> Any of the needs assessment exercises in 3A may also reveal service needs.

- Consider if you are aware of sources of well-informed and impartial careers support for your trainee and other learners, including careers information, guidance and counselling. Find out from professional bodies, deaneries, workforce development confederations, universities etc., if there are sources of which you are currently unaware.
- Reflect on whether you are aware of available courses for trainees and learners in Jayne's speciality areas.
- Organise a force-field analysis exercise in your practice or department to consider the scope and depth of education and training currently provided or available to trainees and other learners.

## Stage 4: Make and carry out a learning and action plan

- Discuss how to help a trainee in Jayne's situation with other teachers at a peer support meeting or workshop for advancing teaching skills.
- Visit a workplace where the induction process is recognised by others as best practice and learn about the components of a good induction and how that might be evaluated.

- Read up on 'how to do' a training needs analysis from a suitable publication obtained from the human resources department or local educational department, or after a search of the literature.
- Find out what resources are available to support Jayne's further professional development or career development from NHS management locally. For example, could Jayne take study leave if she wished and you supported her application?

### Stage 5: Document your learning, competence, performance and standards of service delivery

- Obtain a report of the training needs analysis.
- Compile a checklist for ideal induction that can be individualised according to the needs and circumstances of future learners.
- Keep a database of resources available for supporting education and training and careers development of all kinds of trainees likely to be placed with you.
- Record the force-field analysis.
- You might include a copy of an example past examination paper and your and Jayne's discussion about how her performance might have fallen short. The action plan for those areas of weakness will be an essential part of Jayne's professional development portfolio as well.

---

**Box 11.8:**   Case study continued

Jayne did recover from her disappointment fairly soon with your encouragement. She did consult a careers guidance adviser but this confirmed her enthusiasm for her speciality area and her determination to progress her career in that field. With some dedicated study time and the helpful approach listed above, she passed her speciality examination at the next attempt.

---

# Example cycle of evidence 11.3

- Focus: communication skills
- Other relevant focus: teamworking

---

**Box 11.9:** Case study – encouraging a reluctant team member

Kim has problems working in a team. Others see her as withdrawn, aloof and impersonal. When you confront her with recent remarks from the nurses that they resent the way that she does not adhere to the team protocols, she admits to you that she has always had difficulties relating to a group and prefers a one-to-one situation. She had not realised that other team members thought that she was not fitting in. You discuss how she might communicate better with the rest of the team and improve her teamworking.

---

This is just an example. Keep your task simple. You could choose three or four cycles of evidence to demonstrate your competence as a teacher each year.

*Stage 1: Select your aspirations for good practice*

The excellent healthcare teacher:

- enables learners to recognise and overcome problem areas of working about which they were previously unaware.

*Stage 2: Set the standards for your outcomes*

---

Outcomes might include:

- a tutorial plan
- mastery of a new skill as a teacher
- a teaching strategy that is implemented
- learner feedback
- evaluation of teaching programmes.

---

- Demonstrate good teamworking (*see* page 31).

## Stage 3A: Identify your learning needs

- Conduct a self-appraisal of the extent and nature of teamworking.
- Draw a diagram of the Johari Window (*see* Figure 11.1) and work out how you and Kim relate to it concerning her teamworking skills and insights into related issues. Reflect on the categories with which her behaviour fits (*see* pages 168–9).
- Audit key areas of team members' delivery of clinical care to find out the extent to which each member is providing care to the agreed standards, and check that patients are not at risk from poor teamworking.

## Stage 3B: Identify your service needs

> Any of the needs assessment exercises in 3A may also reveal service needs.

- Find out by direct enquiry the extent to which team members share a clear picture of the organisation's goals and priorities.
- Review your own and learners' PDPs to examine links with the professional development plan of all the team colleagues.
- Carry out a force-field analysis of positive drivers and restraining factors in relation to attainment of a good teamworking culture.
- Undergo an external review relating to teamworking by an accrediting body such as Investors in People or the RCGP's Quality Team Development.

## Stage 4: Make and carry out a learning and action plan

- Read up about the effects of feedback on the Johari Window model and how to apply it in giving Kim feedback.[3]
- Compare the teamworking in your own organisation with examples of best practice.
- Share the problem with other colleagues (but protecting Kim's identity as far as possible) such as your CPD tutor, line managers or training leads.

## Stage 5: Document your learning, competence, performance and standards of service delivery

- Conduct a self-appraisal of the extent of teamworking and keep objective evidence such as an audit of clinical care, picking out each team member's contribution.
- Keep a diagram of the Johari Window model when Kim's problem with teamworking is first identified, and another diagram after the learning session to discuss it and set up the development plan.

- Conduct a force-field analysis about the extent and nature of teamworking and the plan to build and sustain teamworking.
- Keep an external review report containing the identified weaknesses, the plan to address these weaknesses and the progress made.

---

**Box 11.10:**   Case study continued

The audits of delivery of care show that Kim is working to agreed care protocols, and it is more a matter of perception and poor communication that Kim is not fitting in. The insights from the discussion about teamworking and feedback about her personal style help Kim to realise she must make an effort to overcome her natural diffidence about interacting with others in the team, for the sake of good teamworking in delivering patient care.

---

# References

1   Luft J (1970) *Group Processes: an introduction to group dynamics.* National Press Books, Palo Alto, CA.

2   Pendleton D, Schofield T, Tate P and Havelock P (2003) *The New Consultation. Developing doctor–patient communication.* Oxford University Press, Oxford.

3   Chambers R, Wakley G, Iqbal Z and Field S (2002) *Prescription for Learning: techniques, games and activities.* Radcliffe Medical Press, Oxford.

# 12

# Providing supervision and support

The first part of this chapter describes different supervisory or support roles and in the second, teaching and supporting learners with special needs and aspects of pastoral care are considered.

*Mentoring* is: 'the process by which an experienced, highly regarded, empathic person (the mentor) guides another individual (the mentee) in the development and re-examination of their own ideas, learning and personal and professional development'.[1]

A *'buddy'* is someone in a similar situation to you with whom you have a reciprocal relationship, who gives you unconditional peer support. Both buddies should be on equal terms and have a mutual regard for each other's opinion. Each should trust the other to preserve confidentiality about the issues discussed.

*An educational supervisor* works with the learner to develop and facilitate an educational plan that addresses their educational needs. An educational supervisor should:

- meet with the learner early in the post and help with the induction to the post
- agree aims and objectives for learning in the post
- construct the learning agreement with the learner
- give feedback on progress to the learner
- discuss career aims and the training programme
- assess the learner at the end of the post on their learning objectives
- give feedback to the teacher on the training posts and programmes (if appropriate).

*A careers counsellor* is a specialised role, helping people to recognise and utilise their resources to manage career-related problems and make career-related decisions.

People need careers counselling when:

- they are dissatisfied with their current job or career prospects
- they seem unable to solve their career dilemma by themselves although they do usually have the resources to do so

- their thinking is clouded about their career and they need to talk things through with someone who is independent and non-judgemental
- they are not responding to the usual motivators at work
- they seem unaware of the consequences of their poor performance or behaviour at work
- they are engaging in self-deprecating behaviour at work
- they are unaware of their talents and strengths at work.

*Coaching* involves a combination of psychology, business and communication skills. It consists of a partnership between coach and 'client' to clarify the client's goals for work and life and plan how to achieve those goals. A good coach will be a successful motivator, be very supportive, establish a good rapport with the person being coached, be able to give constructive feedback and set clear objectives.

# Potential for role conflict

Some of the responsibilities we have as we act in these, and other, different capacities to the same student might overlap. Sometimes qualities useful to us in one role can be used to great advantage in another. Career counsellor and appraiser might be one such area.

Potentially however there is a risk of conflict of interest. For example, how does our responsibility as line manager for a learner interact with the responsibility as their educational supervisor? Might we want, as a line manager responsible for the safe running of the department, to keep a junior away from patients for the time being – while as educational supervisor realise that supervised experience is what she or he needs to improve?

You can tell if things are not working out if any of the features in the list below apply:

- the mentor talks non-stop
- one of two buddies does not want to meet up any more
- the trainee is not able to confide in his educational supervisor because he knows he will soon be wanting a reference
- a supervisor puts service needs consistently above an individual's training needs
- the careers counsellor is fond of telling his or her clients how he or she managed his or her own career
- the coach undermines others' self-confidence and self-esteem.

Appendix 1 gives an example of the mix of roles and responsibilities required to maintain a general dental practice (GDP) vocational training post in one deanery.

# Adapting your teaching style and habits for learners with disabilities

An effective teacher adapts their delivery to meet the needs of their students. This can be quite a challenge when those students have physical disabilities or mental ill-health (*see* Table 12.1).

**Table 12.1:** Examples of types of disabilities that students may have that could affect their learning

| Type of disability | Possible effects on learning | Possible solutions to minimising disability |
|---|---|---|
| Blindness/visual impairment | Cannot read audiovisual aids<br>Social isolation<br>Disorientated<br>Limited contact with other students<br>Loss of confidence – feels vulnerable<br>May feel 'stupid' | Convert learning materials to Braille by technology<br>Teacher sends learning materials to student by email prior to session to be blown up to huge font size<br>Ensure good lighting in teaching room |
| Deafness/hearing impairment | Cannot hear teacher<br>Similar effects of isolation as for visual impairment<br>Frustration<br>Self-conscious/embarrassed | Teacher stands so that deaf student can lip read<br>Buddy or mentor helps student in teaching session<br>Eliminate background noise |
| Dyslexia | Slower handwriting that may contain grammatical mistakes – impedes response in examinations | Student uses computer for written work when possible<br>Special arrangements for examinations |
| Cancer and equivalent serious illness | Time off for treatment or during relapse – may miss teaching sessions or examinations<br>Pain and other symptoms may interfere with learning | Teacher provides work for student when ill and helps with catching up if possible |
| Immobility e.g. wheelchair bound, fractured leg | Immobility may limit practical work<br>Difficulty accessing resources, teaching rooms, facilities or toilets<br>May feel a 'burden'<br>Loss of confidence if student does not feel on equal terms with able students | Check intended teaching rooms and resources are accessible and swap location if not<br>Provide ramps, disabled car parking |

*continued overleaf*

**Table 12.1:** *continued*

| Type of disability | Possible effects on learning | Possible solutions to minimising disability |
|---|---|---|
| Depression | Lack of concentration Social isolation makes networking difficult Loss of confidence | Teacher is supportive and encouraging |
| Anxiety, stress | Panic attacks Lack of concentration Apprehensive | Teacher is encouraging, breaking down learning into chunks so not overwhelming |
| Claustrophobia, agoraphobia | Panic attacks Lack of concentration | Teacher allows student to sit or stand where they are comfortable |
| Speech impediment | Many of the above effects, relating to loss of confidence Limited ability or wish to make oral presentations, ask questions | Teacher provides alternatives to oral presentation and asks student on a one-to-one basis if they have questions |
| Epilepsy – poorly controlled | Unpredictable fit will disrupt teaching session for student and others Feeling self-conscious and vulnerable | Teacher learns how to react appropriately to an epileptic attack |
| Limited hand function e.g. arthritis, trauma | Limited ability to undertake practical work, use computer, write | Teacher tries to provide alternative methods of learning and assessment |

Many of these disabilities will have common effects on students – who can feel self-conscious and vulnerable because they are different from other students. They may fear being a 'burden' to the teacher and other students and be reluctant to ask for help. They will need help and encouragement to be able to network with the others in small groups, or to participate in plenary sessions.

Good teachers are also aware of the negative effects learners may perceive in being 'singled out' for special attention. It requires great sensitivity to address difference without making it more of a barrier.[2]

You should brush up your knowledge of the Disability Discrimination Act (1995), which covers training and development.

# Pastoral care

It is clear that learners come to us not only with their own personalities and dispositions but their hopes and aspirations, past experiences and backgrounds, worries, responsibilities and anxieties. Very often it will not be appropriate or necessary to make enquiries into any of these factors but some teaching relationships can be affected by such 'outside' factors and some learners find these factors get in the way of learning.

The special context of healthcare teaching, dealing as it does with factors influencing health, life and death, has the potential to be especially challenging for our learners. They may have to learn to deal with the sights, smells and sounds of pain, disease and death, difficult situations such as disturbed or abusive patients, variations in socio-economic background of patients, and health inequalities that frustrate and surprise them. Some might be embarrassed or distressed by the difference between their relative affluence and the circumstances of some patients. They may experience situations that mimic painful times in their own life such as the death of a parent or a child.

In addition they will be working in a sensitive environment where mistakes can have overwhelming consequences. They need to learn how to cope with responsibility for their decisions, to take measured risks without being foolhardy or paralysed by fear of the consequences.

The role of the learner in a healthcare setting can be uncomfortable for these and many other reasons and at the same time their behaviour and performance are under constant surveillance for what they show about their competence and their character.

The factors shown in Box 12.1 may help to ensure that learners cope with all these sources of anxiety, and that they know where to turn when they are not.[3]

---

**Box 12.1:**   Providing support and supervision[3]

- Ensure that students feel able to seek help without loss of confidence or self-esteem by attending to the way questions are answered and requests for support are handled.
- Foster feelings of self-confidence with praise and constructive feedback.
- Try to build in an element of choice about cases they are exposed to.
- Be aware of the power of role modelling as a way to reinforce desired behaviours.
- Encourage self-monitoring and evaluation of performance.
- Be prepared to listen to, and learn from, the experiences that students describe.
- Give learners time to reflect on what has happened and is happening, promote discussion about patient care and always allow time to debrief following significant events.
- Allow learners to make mistakes but be aware of your power to manipulate events to allow success.
- Show confidence in the abilities of your learners; reinforce their expectation of success.

---

We need to be aware of, and prepared to signpost the way to, occupational health services, counsellors, Relate, Citizens Advice Bureaux, the university or hospital chaplain or other sources of advice and support as appropriate.

# Collecting data to demonstrate your learning, competence, performance and standards of service delivery

## Example cycle of evidence 12.1

- Focus: providing supervision and support

---

**Box 12.2:**   Case study – teaching and supporting learners with disabilities

As a trainer, Amir is responsible for cohorts of students who rotate through his speciality area with a different group attending every four weeks. He prides himself on addressing learners' needs and providing training in an equitable way, whether or not students have a disability or any other impediment to learning. He has been responsible for students with dyslexia, some who are visually impaired, others with mobility problems who are wheelchair bound and others with mental health problems such as depression. Colleagues know of his special interest and expertise and contact him for advice if they have students with disabilities.

---

This is just an example. Keep your task simple. You could choose three or four cycles of evidence to demonstrate your competence as a teacher each year.

*Stage 1: Select your aspirations for good practice*

The excellent healthcare teacher:

- takes care not to disadvantage students with special needs due to their physical or mental disabilities.

## *Stage 2: Set the standards for your outcomes*

Outcomes might include:

- a tutorial plan
- mastery of a new skill as a teacher
- a teaching strategy that is implemented
- learner feedback
- evaluation of teaching programmes.

- Effective induction and training of teachers in relation to equity and diversity to accommodate the needs of learners with disabilities.
- An environment that enables students with disabilities to learn on equal terms with those without disabilities as far as is practicable.

## *Stage 3A: Identify your learning needs*

- Read through Table 12.1. Consider how to reproduce in your teaching setting the possible solutions to minimising the impact of a student's disability. Discuss with other teaching colleagues to elicit their ideas for possible solutions or their experiences of what works in practice.
- Talk to one or more students with different types of disability whom you or others have taught, to hear more about their experiences of you or others as teachers, and what you might have done to improve their opportunities for learning.
- Find out if the educational organisation you work with has guidance for handling students with disabilities or making allowances for their disability in assessment.

## *Stage 3B: Identify your service needs*

Any of the needs assessment exercises in 3A may also reveal service needs.

- Meet with students' representatives or invite other help in identifying problems that students with disabilities are likely to encounter.
- Audit any aspect of the structure or process of the teaching or learning activities to find out if students with disabilities are disadvantaged (e.g. access to postgraduate education rooms or resources, insufficient sign-posting or lighting). Discuss with students whether there are barriers that

the service could overcome or additional training that might help, for example in assertiveness skills.

## Stage 4: Make and carry out a learning and action plan

- Attend activities of a voluntary group dedicated to championing disability in order to understand the issues better, knowing that those with disabilities may have low expectations of help and be reluctant to ask for special treatment. Learn from them about equipment that might minimise disability e.g. technological solutions to visual and hearing impairments.
- Run a seminar for other teachers on minimising the impact of students' disabilities on their learning and career expectations. Feed information about the need for resources back to management as appropriate.
- Read reports from initiatives that have helped disabled people in working and learning. Derive information about contact details and sources of help so that you can advise on entitlement to benefits and the nature of practical help available.[4]

## Stage 5: Document your learning, competence, performance and standards of service delivery

- Keep copies of documents or tools that facilitate teaching those with disabilities.
- Retain notes or feedback from students with different disabilities, giving personal perspectives of what works and is desired, what works but creates embarrassment, what does not work, etc.
- Collect a range of helpful literature from a voluntary group championing the rights of disabled people in working and learning.

---

**Box 12.3:**   Case study continued

Amir's advocacy of students with disabilities was taken up as a development theme by the human resources department of his trust who extended the facilitatory approach to staff working in the organisation as well.

---

# Example cycle of evidence 12.2

- Focus: mentoring

---

**Box 12.4:** Case study – mentoring

You have just volunteered to be a mentor because you have gained so much from being mentored yourself. You had a mentor for the first year after you qualified and again more recently. The first relationship worked well and your mentor was non-judgemental, empathetic, open and approachable. The second mentor used to unload his own problems at the end of each mentoring session and you were glad when he explained that with the changes in NHS working he just had not got time to carry on. You thought this was an excuse to save face because it was obvious that the relationship was not working. You resolve to be as good as your first mentor.

---

This is just an example. Keep your task simple. You could choose three or four cycles of evidence to demonstrate your competence as a teacher each year.

*Stage 1: Select your aspirations for good practice*

The excellent healthcare mentor:

- establishes an honest and trustworthy relationship with the person being mentored
- guides the person being mentored to take up personal, professional and career development opportunities.

*Stage 2: Set the standards for your outcomes*

---

Outcomes might include:

- a tutorial plan
- mastery of a new skill as a teacher
- a teaching strategy that is implemented
- learner feedback
- evaluation of teaching programmes.

---

- Establish a good and open relationship between both parties, by adopting formative and supportive roles.
- The person being mentored gains new insights and perspectives and enjoys being challenged to change.

## *Stage 3A: Identify your learning needs*

If you have not started out as a mentor and are considering it:

- reflect on the good qualities of a mentor and check the extent to which you already have those qualities by discussion with a trusted colleague or friend. Ask them if they would provide a reference for you to support your application to be a mentor, as an exercise for you to read and consider their perspectives
- talk to others who are mentors: what is the time commitment, how do they deal with interpersonal conflicts, how long has the mentoring relationship lasted, how do they defuse the 'halo' effect if it happens, are they paid and if not can the meetings be carried out in non-work time? Reflect on whether you can create that spare time and maintain the degree of commitment needed over time
- in your discussion with the mentoring lead find out how much training is provided or available, and what ongoing support is arranged
- obtain a job description for the mentor role or ask the mentor lead to write one if none exists; make a judgement if you have sufficient knowledge and skills or training needs.

If you have started as a mentor already:

- work out a system with the lead for recruiting and supporting mentors. Ask the current person being mentored for their honest appraisal of your strengths and weaknesses as a mentor
- participate in role play exercises at mentor training and support sessions and receive peer feedback on your attitudes and responses.

## *Stage 3B: Identify your service needs*

> Any of the needs assessment exercises in 3A may also reveal service needs.

- Ask the lead for recruiting mentors for anonymised feedback from the people who have been mentored.

## Stage 4: Make and carry out a learning and action plan

- Attend a training workshop for new or potential mentors.
- Talk to established mentors and anyone who tells you that they are being or have been mentored. Find out what it is they most value about the relationship.
- Read widely about the history and practice of mentoring in health settings and other public or commercial sectors.[1,5,6]
- Learn how to record and use informal feedback by discussion with others (or read Chapter 7).

## Stage 5: Document your learning, competence, performance and standards of service delivery

- Keep a job description for the mentor role with written reflections as to your knowledge and skills and training needs and how they will or have been met.
- Obtain feedback from the person being mentored or from those mentored in the past.
- Make notes of key points and what you have learnt from recommended reading material.
- Retain a copy of the contract for mentoring.

---

**Box 12.5:** Case study continued

You attend the initial training workshop and follow-up session six months later, once the mentoring is under way. You really gel with your new person being mentored, who would be surprised to know that she is your first person being mentored. She particularly benefits from your skills at challenging her perceptions and perspectives and goes on to represent staff in strategic working groups, which she would not have previously dared to do.

---

# Example cycle of evidence 12.3

- Focus: clinical supervision

---

**Box 12.6:** Case study – clinical supervision

Mary organises group clinical supervision for the G and H grade district nurses and health visitors whom she line manages in her trust. Practice nurses do not participate although they have been invited to join. Mary wants to let the practice nurses know more about what clinical supervision entails and its benefits, to promote a reflective culture among nurses sited in general practice settings.

---

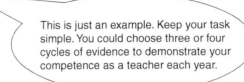

This is just an example. Keep your task simple. You could choose three or four cycles of evidence to demonstrate your competence as a teacher each year.

## Stage 1: Select your aspirations for good practice

The excellent clinical supervisor:

- provides a supportive and challenging role that enables the practitioner being supervised to reflect on their performance in a positive way.

## Stage 2: Set the standards for your outcomes

Outcomes might include:

- a tutorial plan
- mastery of a new skill as a teacher
- a teaching strategy that is implemented
- learner feedback
- evaluation of teaching programmes.

- Establish a well-functioning model of clinical supervision, which provides one-to-one or group clinical supervision depending on practitioners' needs and preferences.

## Stage 3A: Identify your learning needs

- Read up in a variety of texts about the concept of clinical supervision and how it is interpreted and implemented at local level.[7] Read about one-to-one, group and live supervision (supervisor observes practitioner's clinical skills in the workplace) and reflect on the advantages of each approach.
- Obtain personal anonymised feedback from practitioners being supervised about satisfaction and concerns relating to the structure, process and outcomes of the clinical supervision arrangements and your supervisory input.

## Stage 3B: Identify your service needs

Any of the needs assessment exercises in 3A may also reveal service needs.

- Find out what training, protected time and support is available for those providing clinical supervision. Find out what resources are available for funding costs of meetings and development needs emerging from clinical supervision sessions.
- Determine whether the practice, directorate or trust addresses practitioners' learning and support needs emerging from clinical supervision, and how that influences their personal or professional development plans. Discover the availability and accessibility of support resources, e.g. occupational health services, human resources advice, health and safety expertise.
- Undertake a SWOT analysis of clinical supervision arrangements and determine the weaknesses and opportunities that should be tackled.

## Stage 4: Make and carry out a learning and action plan

- Individual practitioners might clarify their roles and responsibilities relating to needs and concerns emerging from clinical supervision.
- Carry out reading as in Stage 3A.[7]
- In the new role as clinical supervisor, discuss with your own clinical supervisor likely problems that may arise and options for response.
- Write about the experience to share good practice. Perhaps contribute to a nurse forum newsletter describing the typical content and advantages of clinical supervision, and citing much of the information gleaned from activities in section 3B.

## Stage 5: Document your learning, competence, performance and standards of service delivery

- Note key points from standard texts about clinical supervision.
- Keep a record of the SWOT analysis.
- Write reflections from discussions with clinical supervisor colleagues.
- Compile a checklist of needs identified by those practitioners being supervised matched with the needs actually met by the organisation.

---

**Box 12.7:**   Case study continued

The article about clinical supervision, prominently included in the newsletter disseminated to all primary care nurses by the nurse forum, engages the interest of several practice nurses. They come along as a trio to the clinical supervision group of district nurses, enjoy the session and attend regularly. Eventually there is so much interest by word of mouth that a separate clinical supervision group is created.

---

# References

1   Standing Committee on Postgraduate Medical and Dental Education (1998) *An Enquiry into Mentoring: supporting doctors and dentists at work.* Standing Committee on Postgraduate Medical and Dental Education, London.

2   Halstead JA (1998) Teaching students with special needs. In: DM Billings and JA Jalstead (eds) *Teaching in Nursing: a guide for faculty.* WB Saunders, Philadelphia.

3   Stuart C (2003) *Assessment, Supervision and Support in Clinical Practice. A guide for nurses, midwives and other health professionals.* Churchill Livingstone, London.

4   Roulstone A, Gradwell L, Price J and Child L (2003) *How Disabled People Manage in the Workplace.* Joseph Rowntree Foundation, London. www.jrf.org.uk.

5   Freeman R (1998) *Mentoring in General Practice.* Butterworth-Heinemann, Woburn.

6   Carmin CN (1988) Issues on research in mentoring: definitional and methodological. *International Journal of Mentoring.* **2**: 9–13.

7   Butterworth T, Faugier J and Burnard P (eds) (1998) *Clinical Supervision and Mentorship in Nursing.* Nelson Thornes, Cheltenham.

# Further reading

*   British Medical Association (1996) *Guidelines for the Provision of Careers Services for Doctors.* British Medical Association, London.
*   BMJ Career Focus series at www.bmj.com.
*   Chambers R, Mohanna K and Field S (2000) *Opportunities and Options in Medical Careers.* Radcliffe Medical Press, Oxford.
*   Francis D (1994) *Managing your own Career.* HarperCollins, London.
*   Freeman R (1996) Mentoring in general practice. *Education for General Practice.* **7**: 112–17.
*   Gupta R (1998) *Handbook on Mentoring and Career Counselling for Doctors.* Overseas Doctors Association, Lancashire.
*   Handy C (1995) *The Age of Unreason.* Arrow Business Books, London.
*   Schein E (1990) *Career Anchors: discovering your real needs.* Pfeiffer and Company, Oxford.
*   Schein E (1990) *Career Anchors: trainer's manual.* Pfeiffer and Company, Oxford.
*   Ward C and Eccles S (2001) *So You Want to be a Brain Surgeon? A medical careers guide* (2e). Oxford Medical Publications, Oxford.

# APPENDIX 1

## Example of ten requirements for general dental practice vocational training posts in the West Midlands Deanery

1  *Programme director*: each vocational dental practitioner (VDP) must have an approved named GDP trainer who accepts responsibility for planning the educational programme and ensuring that the standards set out below are met.

2  *Protected teaching*: at least one hour of protected time within surgery hours will be put aside for a tutorial within a training practice. Ideally the topic for the tutorial will be agreed in advance and suitable arrangements made to identify resources that may be of use. The topics for the tutorials may address educational needs identified by comments made by the VDP in the Professional Development Portfolio. In addition, the VDPs will attend 30 study days based at one of five postgraduate centres in the region. Written assessments of the study day presentations will be completed by the VDP at the end of each session, and this information will be used to monitor the quality of the education delivered, and further refine the study days.

3  *Educational supervision*: each VDP must have a named educational supervisor, usually the GDP trainer, who meets with him/her privately at the start of the training year, and then regularly to clarify career goals, identify learning needs and plan the education accordingly. Information from the vocational training (VT) adviser (course organiser) about the VDP's progress must be provided for these sessions.

4  *Feedback/appraisal/assessment*: all general dental practitioners involved in training VDPs must provide regular informal constructive feedback on both good and poor performance and contribute to appraisal and assessment of the VDP.

5  *Induction*: at the beginning of the training year, all VDPs must participate in an induction programme designed to familiarise them with the practice in general, local aspects of dental primary care and the deanery educational

organisation. Written information on the dental practice, timetables and other arrangements must be provided.

6   *Clinical guidelines*: all written guidelines used in the dental practice for common clinical conditions must be available to the VDP. These should be evidence based and subject to audit.

7   *Senior cover*: immediate advice from a GDP member (normally the trainer or a senior GDP within the practice) must be available to the VDP. The approved trainer must be coincident in the practice with the VDP on at least three days per week.

8   *Clinical activity*: all VDPs must be exposed to an appropriate level of clinical activity to his/her stage of educational development, for the achievement of educational objectives. By the end of training, the VDP should be able to undertake an appropriate GDP workload.

9   *Inappropriate tasks*: no VDP should be expected to perform work for which he/she is inadequately trained, or which is of no relevance to his/her educational objectives.

10   *Study leave*: VDPs must be allowed to attend courses appropriate to their educational objectives, agreed with their trainer and course organiser within the limits set by the postgraduate dean.

# Index

T - #1041 - 101024 - C0 - 244/170/14 - PB - 9781857756074 - Gloss Lamination